D1594388

Aniridia and WAGR Syndrome

ANIRIDIA AND WAGR SYNDROME

A Guide for Patients and Families

Edited by

Jill Ann Nerby and Jessica J. Otis

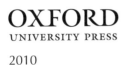

OXFORD

UNIVERSITY PRESS

2010

OXFORD
UNIVERSITY PRESS

Oxford University Press, Inc., publishes works that further
Oxford University's objective of excellence
in research, scholarship, and education.

Oxford   New York
Auckland   Cape Town   Dar es Salaam   Hong Kong   Karachi
Kuala Lumpur   Madrid   Melbourne   Mexico City   Nairobi
New Delhi   Shanghai   Taipei   Toronto

With offices in
Argentina   Austria   Brazil   Chile   Czech Republic   France   Greece
Guatemala   Hungary   Italy   Japan   Poland   Portugal   Singapore
South Korea   Switzerland   Thailand   Turkey   Ukraine   Vietnam

Published by Oxford University Press, Inc.
198 Madison Avenue, New York, New York 10016

www.oup.com

Oxford is a registered trademark of Oxford University Press

Library of Congress Cataloging-in-Publication Data
Aniridia and WAGR syndrome : a guide for patients and families / edited
by Jill Ann Nerby and Jessica J. Otis.
p.   cm.
Includes bibliographical references and index.
ISBN 978-0-19-538930-2
1. Iris (Eye)—Diseases—Popular works.   2. Genetic disorders—Popular works.
3. Syndromes—Popular works.   I. Nerby, Jill Ann.   II. Otis, Jessica J.
RE350.A55 2009
617.7′2—dc22

2009027531

9   8   7   6   5   4   3   2   1

Printed in the United States of America
on acid-free paper

Thank you to all the doctors and contributors to this book. Without you it never would've been written. Together, we would like to dedicate this book to our fellow aniridics. Believe it you can achieve it.

I dedicate this book to my parents, Dennis and Sue, my grandparents Jane and Larry, and my son, Michael, and to all other supportive family members who have loved and helped me throughout my life.

—Jill Ann Nerby
Founder of Aniridia Foundation International

I dedicate this book to my husband, Reid, my son, Lucas, my parents, Eric and Judy, and my "twin," Tura. Without your love and support my dreams never would've come true. Thank you for always being there for me. I am truly grateful to have all of you in my life. Additionally, I would like to dedicate this book to the family who inspired me to do a book to help others with aniridia, the Siciliano family. Thank you for being my inspiration.

—Jessica J. Otis
Editor, *Eye On Aniridia*

Preface

At this time you may have several questions and concerns about aniridia, or perhaps WAGR syndrome. If your child has just been diagnosed with aniridia, or if he or she has just been diagnosed with WAGR Syndrome, you are probably experiencing many different feelings—sadness, anxiety, anger, confusion, and so on. You are not alone. Other parents have felt the same way and have had the same questions. It is very normal to have questions and to feel these emotions.

In 1976, at the age of three months, I was diagnosed with sporadic (not inherited) aniridia and horizontal nystagmus. At that time, my parents had many questions, but could not find many answers. At first they were told I would be completely blind and would not able to attend public school; however, as I grew up, they began to see how wrong the first doctor was in his diagnosis. I (and others with visual impairments) can do many things a person with "normal" vision can do. What can I do that you can do? Well, honestly, a lot of things. For example, I was able to get my driver's license when not many people thought I could do it. Now, please know that not many people with aniridia are able to get a driver's license. I am one of the very few who have gotten one. When I was younger, I wanted it to have more independence, since my small hometown did not have public transportation. But now I only want it in case of emergencies, because honestly I don't enjoy driving. It can be very stressful, and I'd rather let my husband drive. The point to my story is that there is hope for you and your child to have a good life. All you need to do is to believe it.

Many of you may feel like it was your fault that your child was born with aniridia or WAGR syndrome. Many parents feel this way, but please do not blame yourself. In the beginning, my mom blamed herself for my eye condition when there was nothing she could have done. Years later she told the story of how she realized I was given to her for a reason. She says I was five months old when she took my brother and me to see Santa Claus at the mall. While standing in line she saw the most precious little four-year-old girl she'd ever seen. The girl was begging her mother to let her go see Santa. The mother brushed her away like an insect and told her she "didn't have time for such a stupid thing." At that moment my mom felt horrible that this little girl had a mother who would treat her that way. My mom thought, "At least Jessica won't have a mother like that." At first my mom also thought she wasn't strong enough to be a good enough mother to me, but after this experience she realized I was given to her for a reason. She realized she was meant to be my mother to help me become the woman I am today.

While growing up, I never blamed my parents for my eye condition. There was nothing they did wrong. The same goes for you: you did nothing wrong. My parents never could have known it was going to happen. Looking back at my life and all I've experienced, I've come to realize that I was given aniridia and nystagmus so that I can help others see that being visually impaired can be challenging, but isn't always the worst thing that can happen to us. I may not be perfect in the eyes of society, but neither is anyone else. It took me a very long time to realize this and to accept myself for the way I am, especially since growing up was hard at times.

Which brings us to one reason why we are doing this book. This book is needed and long overdue. In it we want to show those affected by aniridia or those affected by WAGR syndrome that they are not alone. There are others out there who can help you through the difficult times. Just by doing this book, I have met so many great people who are affected by aniridia. From them, I learned that each of us has gone through many similar things. It has helped to hear how they dealt with certain situations, and that I'm not alone. That is why Aniridia Foundation International (AFI) is so important to those affected by aniridia. It brings us together so we can support one another, and no one has to go through anything alone. I just wish my parents could have had a support group like Aniridia Foundation International when I was growing up, so they could have had the wonderful information and support it provides. This is why we've put together the most recent medical information, the history of Aniridia Foundation International and how it can help you, other resources of support and information, and personal stories from others affected by aniridia or WAGR syndrome.

Our goal is that this book will help others affected by aniridia and WAGR Syndrome; and enlighten and educate the public. Most of all, we hope it inspires and gives you hope that you and your child can have a good life, even if it can be a challenging life. And that together we can make a difference. Take our hands, Walk with us, Share our dreams, Help us make a miracle!

—Jessica J. Otis

Contents

About the Authors

Lama A. Al-Aswad, M.D.

Dr. Al-Aswad is on the Aniridia Foundation International's medical advisory board, and is an invaluable asset to the foundation. She is an assistant professor of clinical ophthalmology in the glaucoma division of the Edward S. Harkness Eye Institute, Columbia University College of Physicians and Surgeons. She is a very caring and passionate doctor who enjoys helping others. She is extremely interested in the research of antimetabolite use in glaucoma, ocular blood flow in glaucoma, and glaucoma drainage implants. Her clinical interests are complicated glaucoma, normal tension glaucoma, congenital and pediatric glaucoma, glaucoma aqueous shunt surgery, and filtration surgery with antimetabolite. Dr. Al-Aswad is a member of the American Academy of Ophthalmology, the Association for Research in Vision and Ophthalmology (ARVO), the New York State Ophthalmological Society, the American Glaucoma Society, the Chandlear-Grant Glaucoma Society, the New York Ophthalmological Society, and the New York Glaucoma Society. She is also the author of several papers, abstracts, and chapters. With Dr. Peter Netland, she wrote the chapter "Laser Treatment in Glaucoma" in *Clinical Guide to Glaucoma Management*.

Jennifer K. Bulmann, O.D., F.A.A.O.

Dr. Bulmann recieved her O.D. at Illinois College of Optometry in 1998. She completed her residency in Geriatric and Rehabilitative Optometry at the Birmingham VA Medical Center in Birmingham, Alabama, in 2000. She has research interest in low vision. Dr. Bulmann is a member of the American Optometric Association, the West Tennessee Optometric Society and a fellow in the American Academy of Optometry. She is also a board member of MidSouth Chapter of the Foundation Fighting Blindness. Dr. Bulmann is the low vision optometrist at the Memphis VA Medical Center and adjunct professor at the Southern College of Optometry in Memphis, Tennessee. In 2002, Dr. Bulmann won the American Optometric Foundation (AOF) Poster Award at Southern Education Congress of Optometry (SECO) International, and in 1998, she won the Low Vision Rehabilitation Service award.

Mayank Gupta, M.D.

Dr. Mayank Gupta is a post-doctorate fellow at the University of Illinois, Chicago, in the ophthalmology department and visual sciences. Dr. Gupta is a member of the Medical Council of India and the General Medical Council in England. In addition, he has published several works, including the book "Pathology of Glaucoma" in *Principle and Practice of Ophthalmology* (3rd ed., 2007) and the article "Benefit and means of good control and monitoring of diabetes mellitus" in *Folia Pharmacologica*. Currently, Dr. Gupta is researching the development of a novel slit lamp-based femtosecond laser delivery system for laser trabecular ablation in glaucoma.

Edward J. Holland, M.D.

Dr. Edward Holland is the Director, Cornea Services at the Cincinnati Eye Institute. His clinical interests include ocular surface transplantation, corneal transplantation, cataract surgery, and refractive surgery. Dr. Holland has extensive expertise in corneal and external diseases, and he has been listed in *Best Doctors in America*. Dr. Holland serves on the Aniridia Foundation International's Executive Board of Directors and Medical Advisory Board. He also serves on the American Academy of Ophthalmology's Board of Trustees and is Secretariat of the Annual Meeting for the American Academy of Ophthalmology. He is chair of the Medical Advisory Board for the Eye Bank Association of America, and serves on the Executive Committee for the American Society of Cataract and Refractive Surgeons. Dr. Holland was named the 2008 Binkhorst lecturer at the American Society of Cataract and Refractive Surgeons meeting. Dr. Holland has written over 100 articles, edited the widely read textbook *Cornea*, and has co-edited the textbook *Ocular Surface Disease: Medical and Surgical Management*. He is a recipient of several awards, including the Paton Society Award in 2002 from the Eye Bank Association of America. Dr. Holland appeared on ABC's reality show *Miracle Workers*, where he performed stem cell and cornea transplants for a man with Steven Johnson's syndrome. These procedures helped restore the man's sight in his left eye after he had been totally blind for twenty-two years. Dr. Holland is a very dedicated doctor who has helped many people, including this book's co-editor, Jill Nerby. She is not only grateful to him for restoring her sight, but for his assistance in fighting blindness by being on the Executive Board of Directors of Aniridia Foundation International.

Alison Krangel

Alison Krangel has sporadic aniridia, glaucoma, nystagmus, ptosis, and corneal pannus. She received a B.A. in psychology: cognitive rehabilitation from West Chester University of Pennsylvania, and a M.S. in clinical health psychology from the Philadelphia College of Osteopathic Medicine. She volunteers her time to the Aniridia Foundation International (AFI) by writing a human issues column in AFI's quarterly members' newsletter, *Eye on Aniridia*. Alison also records each issue of *Eye on Aniridia* on audiocassette for those who choose to receive it on tape.

James D. Lauderdale, Ph.D.

Dr. James D. Lauderdale is an assistant professor in the department of cellular biology at the University of Georgia in Athens, Georgia. Dr. Lauderdale completed his undergraduate education at Alma College, a small liberal arts college in Michigan. He received his doctorate in biology in 1992 from Purdue University under the direction of Dr. Arnie Stein, and completed his postdoctoral work at the University of Michigan. Dr. Lauderdale's first post-doctoral work was with Dr. John Y. Kuwada (1992–1997), and his second was with Dr. Tom Glaser (1997–2000). Since arriving at the University of Georgia, Dr. Lauderdale's laboratory has been investigating the role of limbal stem cells in maintaining the cornea and the mechanisms that control PAX6 expression during eye development. These studies will lead to a better under-standing of aniridia and other related eye defects in humans, and should facilitate the development of therapies that could restore vision or correct vision-related problems. He currently serves on the medical advisory board of Aniridia Foundation International and is a member of several scientific organizations.

Anil K. Mandal, M.D.

Dr. Mandal is the director of the Jasti V. Ramanamma Children's Eye Care Centre, and consultant at the VST Centre for Glaucoma Care. He is a glaucoma specialist with particular experience and interest in developmental glaucoma. He has won several national and international awards, including the Bhatnagar Award for Achievement in Medical Science in 2003. Dr. Mandal has also published several works in premier journals. Currently, Dr. Mandal is focused on researching clinical and genetic components of glaucoma in children and adults. Dr. Mandal would like to acknowledge and thank Harsha B.L. Rao for assisting him in completing the genetics chapter of this book.

Jill Ann Nerby, Aniridia Foundation International Founder and CEO

Jill Nerby was born with sporadic aniridia and congenital glaucoma. She received a bachelor of science degree in biology/psychology with an emphasis in genetics. She then went on to complete two more years of pre-med classes in an effort to go to medical or occupational therapy school; however, she developed corneal pannus and could not complete the pro-gram. In 2001, her experiences with these conditions, as well as her passion to help others, educate the public, and her desire to make a difference in the aniridia population, especially for the children of today and tomorrow, led her to create a 501(c)3 nonprofit organization called the U.S.A. Aniridia

Network. In 2006, it went worldwide as the Aniridia Foundation International. Jill has been an invited speaker at many events, and an exhibitor at medical conferences such as the American Academy of Ophthalmology. She is available for speaking engagements by calling AFI's office. Jill has a son, Michael, who inherited aniridia from her.

Peter A. Netland, M.D., Ph.D.

Dr. Peter Netland serves on the AFI's executive board of directors and medical advisory board. Currently, Dr. Netland is also the Chairman of Ophthalmology at the University of Virginia School of Medicine. Dr. Netland has vast experience with aniridia and glaucoma, and has authored many reviews, reports, and monographs in ophthalmic literature. He coauthored the book *The Pediatric Glaucomas* with Dr. Anil Mandal. Dr. Netland was elected to the American Ophthalmological Society in 2009. He is an outstanding clinician, and has traveled worldwide to perform surgeries and educate physicians. He is an inspiration to all who have the privilege of making his acquaintance. He has an extraordinary list of accomplishments, and just one of them is helping to develop AFI.

Jessica J. Otis

Jessica Jo Otis was born with sporadic aniridia and horizontal nystagmus. She received a B.A. in English (emphasis on creative and practical writing) from Western Michigan University in 1999. She is the editor of Aniridia Foundation International's quarterly members' newsletter, the *Eye on Aniridia*. She has a son, Lucas, who has inherited aniridia and nystagmus from her.

Mark Pishotta, L.P.C., N.C.C.

Mark Pishotta has a private practice and is also a crisis-intervention counselor in Milwaukee, Wisconsin. He is a licensed professional counselor and a nationally certified counselor. Over the past several years, he has worked with and studied several children and adolescents in a variety of settings. He has also worked with children diagnosed with Asperger's disorder, autism, and other developmental disabilities. Mark's past experiences have helped in his knowledge and understanding of children and adolescents.

Harsha B. L. Rao M.S., D.N.B.

Harsha completed his basic medical education at Bangalore Medical College, Bangalore, and his M.S. in ophthalmology from Minto Regional Institute of Ophthalmology, Bangalore. He completed his long-term fellowship in glaucoma from L.V. Prasad Eye Institute (LVPEI) and is presently working as a consultant in VST Glaucoma Centre at LVPEI. His areas of interest include glaucoma diagnostics and decision-making in glaucoma treatment.

Lookjan Riansuwan, M.D.
Dr. Lookjan Riansuwan is a visiting fellow in Glaucoma Research at Edward S. Harkness Eye Institute, Columbia University College of Physicians and Surgeons. She came to the United States from the department of ophthalmology at the Somdej Prapinkloa Naval Hospital in Bangkok, Thailand. Dr. Riansuwan did her ophthalmologic residency at the Ophthalmology Department of the Faculty of Medicine, Siriraj Hospital.

Aniridia and WAGR Syndrome

1

Aniridia, WAGR Syndrome, and Associated Conditions*

LAMA A. AL-ASWAD, LOOKJAN RIANSUWAN, AND
JESSICA J. OTIS

ANIRIDIA AND WAGR SYNDROME

What is Aniridia?

Aniridia (Greek) literally means "absence of iris" (the colored part of the eye); however, this is a misnomer because patients with aniridia always have irises that are rudimentary or not fully developed.

Years ago when this eye condition was given the name "aniridia," it was not known that the name would come to only describe the most physically noticeable aspect of the condition. Today it is known that the lack of iris is only a minor aspect of aniridia, and it does not reflect the more important aspects of aniridia that can cause even more vision loss. Aniridia has been and still is referred to as a "rare" eye condition, even though the eye conditions that make up aniridia are common ones such as glaucoma, cataract, corneal degeneration, and low vision. The "rare" aspect of aniridia is having the combination of these conditions in one individual, affecting his or her vision.

Aniridia is a genetic eye condition that is congenital—that is, it is present from birth—and affects various structures of the eye. It occurs when the gene responsible for eye development, the PAX6 gene (located on the eleventh chromosome), does not function correctly. The result is developmental disorders not only of the iris, but also of the cornea, the angle of the eye, the lens, the retina (sensory part of the eye), and the optic nerve (nerve that carries visual impulse to the brain). The degree of maldevelopment differs from one patient to another. Aniridia is a bilateral disease. The incidence of this condition ranges from one in 40,000 to one in 50,000 births.[1] It

---

*Editor's note: The medical information concerning WAGR Syndrome and other associated conditions in this chapter is constantly being updated and researched. The new associated conditions and WAGR syndrome information was most recently updated in March, 2009.

occurs equally in males and females, and has no racial predilection. Aniridia can be familial or sporadic (occurs spontaneously, not inherited).

Familial Aniridia (87%): The Ocular Manifestations Occur in Isolation

- 85% autosomal dominant
- 2% autosomal recessive has been observed in the rare Gillespie's syndrome, in which aniridia is associated with cerebellar ataxia, structural defects in the cerebellum and other parts of the brain, and mental retardation. Patients with Gillespie syndrome are not predisposed to the development of Wilms' tumor.

Sporadic Aniridia

- (13%), which can be either with or without Wilms' tumor, genitourinary abnormalities, and mental retardation.

CLINICAL MANIFESTATIONS OF ANIRIDIA

Eye manifestations in patients with aniridia include photophobia (light sensitivity), nystagmus (involuntary eye movements), decreased vision, amblyopia (decreased vision without apparent physical defect or disease), strabismus (squint), corneal opacification, glaucoma, lens abnormalities, retinal abnormalities, and optic nerve abnormalities. Many affected patients have a characteristic facial expression with narrowed palpebral fissure (eye opening) and a furrowed brow, which results from photophobia.

Aniridia also occurs as a component of an association of systemic defects such as mental retardation, genital abnormalities, Wilms' tumor (WAGR), and Gillespie syndrome.

CLASSIFICATION OF ANIRIDIA

Aniridia can be classified into three groups, depending on the sporadic or familial inheritance and associated syndrome.[2]

Aniridia Type One (85%)

- Familial aniridia
- Autosomal dominant
- Isolated ocular defect

Aniridia Type Two (13%) (Miller's Syndrome, WAGR)

- Sporadic (non-familial) aniridia
- Deletion or mutation in short arm of chromosome 11
- Associations include:
  - Wilms' tumor of the kidneys (nephroblastoma)
  - Genitourinary abnormalities
  - Mental retardation
  - Craniofacial dysmorphism (anatomical malformation of the skull and face)
  - Hemihypertrophy (a rare condition in which one side of the body seems to grow faster than the other)

Aniridia Type Three (2%) (Gillespie's Syndrome)

- Autosomal recessive aniridia
- Mental retardation, cerebellar ataxia (uncoordinated muscle movement)
- Structural defects in brain and cerebellum (a portion of the base of the brain, which serves to coordinate voluntary movements, posture, and balance, located in the back of the skull)
- Do not develop Wilms' tumor

WHAT IS WAGR SYNDROME?

WAGR is referred to as a "contiguous gene deletion syndrome," and it can affect males or females. This basically means that there is a deletion of a group of genes on chromosome 11 (11p13). In WAGR, the term *11p13* shows the exact location of the affected part of chromosome 11. In WAGR patients, alterations happen most often on chromosome 11p13 during the early development of an embryo or when a sperm or egg is being created. There is also what is called "translocation." This occurs when one of a child's parents carries a rearrangement between two chromosomes that can cause the loss of some genes; while this occurrence is very rare, all parents should nevertheless be aware of the possibility when planning to have a child. Genetic counseling can be done to determine if the patient has a higher risk of having a child with WAGR syndrome. WAGR patients can have eye problems and be at risk for kidney cancer and mental retardation. WAGR patients typically have two or more of the below-listed conditions; some patients can have WAGR but not all of the mentioned conditions. "WAGR" stands for:

- (W)ilms' Tumor
- (A)niridia
- (G)enitourinary problems
- Mental (R)etardation

WAGR syndrome can also be referred to as:

- WAGR Complex
- Wilms' Tumor-Aniridia-Genitourinary Anomalies-Mental Retardation Syndrome
- Wilms' Tumor-Aniridia-Gonadoblastoma-Mental Retardation Syndrome
- Chromosome 11p deletion syndrome
- 11p deletion syndrome[3]

Diagnoses

Typically, when a patient is born with aniridia, genetic testing can be done to check for the 11p13 deletion to determine if the patient has WAGR syndrome or not. One genetic test that is done is called a *chromosome analysis* or *karyotype*. This test can look for the deleted area (11p13). Another test that can find more detail is called *FISH*, done to look for deletions of particular genes on chromosome 11.

Symptoms

The symptoms of WAGR are typically found at birth. In some cases, an enlargement of the baby's kidneys can be seen during a prenatal ultrasound.[4] Aniridia is normally noticed when a child is newborn. For males, genitals and urinary systems problems are apparent when the child is newborn. WAGR patients have a high risk for developing other problems as they mature into adulthood. The problems may affect the kidneys, eyes, testes, or ovaries. Symptoms that occur in WAGR patients can depend on the combination of disorders that the patient has.

Wilms' Tumor

Roughly fifty percent of WAGR patients develop Wilms' tumor. During the first stages of Wilms' tumor there are typically no symptoms; however, some of the first signs of it can be swelling of the abdomen, blood in the urine, loss of appetite, weight loss, lack of energy, or low-grade fever.

Aniridia

In aniridia patients, the iris does not fully develop, thus causing partial or complete absence of the iris. WAGR patients nearly always have aniridia. Aniridia can cause other eye problems in adulthood.

Dry Eye.   "Dry eye" is defined as a tear-film disorder due to tear deficiency or excessive tear evaporation, resulting in ocular surface damage and eye discomfort. The tear film consists of three layers, produced by different specialized cells. Each layer functions differently, and they act as one unit to maintain the integrity of the ocular surface. Abnormalities in one or more of these layers cause instability and deficiency of the tear film. Dry eye associated with aniridia occurs from increased evaporation of the tear film rather than tear deficiency.[5]

Symptoms of dry eye are itching, burning, irritation, redness, blurred vision that improves with blinking, or excessive tearing and increased discomfort after periods of reading, watching TV, or working on the computer.

Treatment depends on the severity of dry eye. In mild to moderate cases, they can use artificial tear supplementation, while more severe cases need additional interventions.

Corneal Defects.   The cornea is the clear, dome-shaped window covering the front of the eye. The abnormal PAX6 gene can cause abnormalities in the cornea. Generally it results in an irregular, inflamed corneal surface and a subsequent opacity of the cornea (corneal pannus) beginning at the periphery and gradually progressing into the central region of the cornea. It can occur as early as two years of age.[6] Since the normal clear cornea function is essential for good vision, abnormal clarity results in decreased vision in patients with aniridia.

The treatment for corneal opacification and pannus with visual loss is corneal transplant surgery; however, the prognosis is guarded because of corneal graft rejection, underlying amblyopia, glaucoma, and other structural abnormalities.

Microcornea is another corneal abnormality that can be associated with aniridia. Microcornea is corneal size that is smaller in diameter than normal. There is no need for treatment in this condition.

It has been reported that aniridia patients have thicker corneas than normal. This will affect the accuracy of the intraocular pressure measurement, especially in glaucoma patients.[7]

Glaucoma.   Glaucoma can occur at any age from infancy to later in life, but aniridia patients who were born with glaucoma are rare. The incidence of developing glaucoma later in childhood ranges from 6% to 75%.[8] Due to the lifelong risk of glaucoma, aniridia patients should have a regular glaucoma assessment.

Treatments of glaucoma consist of medications and surgery. Medical therapy may be successful in the beginning, but most patients will require surgery later.

Lens Abnormalities.   Aniridia can have associated abnormalities of the lenses. These are cataract (lens opacity) and lens subluxation (lens is partially displaced from its normal position).

Cataract develops in 50%–85% of patients, usually during the first two decades of life.[9] If the opacity causes deterioration in visual function, cataract surgery may be required.

Lens subluxation can occur in up to 56% of aniridia patients.[10] It may cause a reduction in vision. Refractive correction can help in this condition. If the lens is subluxated anteriorly and severe enough, it can result in secondary glaucoma, for which surgery is indicated.

Optic Nerve and Foveal Hypoplasia.   The optic nerve carries visual impulses from the eye to the brain. The fovea is a region in the central part of the retina that produces the sharpest vision. Optic nerve and foveal hypoplasia are conditions in which the optic nerve and fovea are not developed completely, resulting in decreased vision and nystagmus (wobbly eyes). There is no correlation between the degree of aniridia and optic nerve and foveal hypoplasia.[11] These conditions are often difficult to detect in patients with aniridia because of the cloudy cornea and cataract; however, it has been estimated that three-fourths of aniridia patients have optic nerve hypoplasia.[12]

There is no treatment to improve the hypoplasia, but visual rehabilitation is very important in this condition.

Nystagmus (Wobbly Eyes).   Nystagmus is an involuntary movement of the eyes. It is present in the majority of aniridia patients and believed to be secondary to foveal and optic nerve hypoplasia. Some patients have a null point, which is the position that has the least eye movement and therefore improves the vision. Some develop a head position that yields the best vision. Parents and teachers can notice this and decide which side of the classroom is the best for the child.

There is no specific treatment for this condition. Glasses and contact lenses do not correct this condition.

Strabismus.   Strabismus (crossed eyes) is a condition in which the patient is unable to align both eyes simultaneously under normal conditions. It is common in patients with aniridia. In some patients the more distinct form is inward turning of the eyes (esotropia).[13]

Early detection and intervention are important in the treatment of strabismus. Careful eye examination should be performed to search for refractive error and amblyopia. Optical correction and occlusion therapy should begin very early to prevent further reduction in visual acuity from amblyopia. After the condition is stabilized and there is still significant eye deviation remaining, surgery is considered as the next step.

Photophobia.   Photophobia is light sensitivity in normal lighting, which makes the child feel uncomfortable. Photophobia sufferers tend to have a typical facial expression and a furrowed brow.[14] In a normal individual, the iris functions like a diaphragm in a camera. It helps control the amount of light entering the eye. Due to underdevelopment of the irises in aniridia patients, there is excessive light entering the eyes, so patients try to close their eyes when exposed to the light. Other causes of photophobia are corneal irregularity and partial opacity or subluxation of lens. To help reduce these symptoms, a person can use tinted glasses and/or hats that shade the sunlight, change residence, and avoid bright outdoor illumination.[15]

Ptosis.   Ptosis is a condition where the eyelid droops from the normal position. In aniridia, ptosis is bilateral and is usually present at birth.[16] Eyelid surgery is the procedure of choice for the correction of ptosis; however, careful evaluation of the degree of ptosis and associated conditions should be performed prior to the consideration of surgery.

Amblyopia.   Amblyopia (derived from the Greek) means "dullness of vision." It is a condition in which the vision is decreased but no cause can be detected during eye examination. In one study, amblyopia occurred in about 37% of patients with aniridia.

Early detection and management is very important. The treatment consists of correcting media opacities, correcting significant refractive errors, encouraging the child to use the amblyopic eye, and monitoring for recurrence of the amblyopia.

Genital and Urinary (GU) Problems

In some cases, problems with the development of genitals can make the sex of a baby (male or female) unclear when it is born. Some of the GU problems in male WAGR patients include testes that have not descended or the urinary tract opening's being not at the tip of the penis but on the shaft instead. Some problems that may be found in female WAGR patients are undeveloped ovaries or malformations of the uterus, fallopian tubes, or vagina. WAGR patients also have a higher risk of gonadoblastoma, which is a cancer of cells that form the testes or ovaries.[17]

Mental Retardation

WAGR patients frequently have developmental delays or mental retardation. The severity of mental retardation varies from patient to patient. It can range from mild to severe mental retardation, although some WAGR patients can have normal intelligence.

Other Symptoms of WAGR Syndrome

Other symptoms of WAGR commonly found are:

- Developmental, behavioral, and/or psychiatric disorders, including autism, attention deficit disorder, obsessive compulsive disorder, anxiety disorders, and depression
- Early-onset obesity and high blood cholesterol levels
- Excessive food intake
- Chronic kidney failure, most often after the age of twelve
- Breathing problems—asthma, pneumonia, and sleep apnea
- Frequent infections of the ears, nose, and throat, especially during infancy and early childhood
- Teeth problems—crowded or uneven
- Problems with muscle tone and strength, especially during infancy and childhood
- Seizure disorder (epilepsy)
- Inflammation of the pancreas (pancreatitis)[18]

Treatment

Treatment for WAGR patients is determined by the specific symptoms in the patient. Regular examinations of WAGR patients can help catch any problem early so treatment may be given promptly.

Wilms' Tumor

Wilms' tumor generally develops between the age of one and three years. It can occur in about 50% of WAGR patients. Many cases of Wilms' tumor have been detected by the age of eight, but in rare cases have occurred later.[19] WAGR patients should have routine renal (kidney) ultrasounds every three months from birth up to age eight. A second way to check on a routine basis is for the child's doctor to feel the child's abdomen for swelling or masses. Continually watching for signs of Wilms' tumor after the age of eight can be done by ultrasounds and/ or keeping an eye out for other symptoms mentioned above. The survival rate of Wilms' tumor patients is very good, depending on appearance of the tumor and stage of the cancer. The treatments for Wilms' tumor can include chemotherapy, radiation therapy, or surgery to remove a kidney.

Aniridia

The goals for an aniridia patient are to keep the patient's vision and the health of the eye stable. This can be done by regularly monitoring the patient's eyes and pressure of the eyes. A person with aniridia should not wear contact lenses because they can damage the cornea, which can cause further problems such as corneal pannus.

Genital and Urinary Problems

Routine evaluations of ovaries and testes development should be done on WAGR patients. To avoid cancer of the gonads, surgery may be done to remove any abdominal gonads. If both gonads are removed, then the patient can be given hormone replacement treatment. If a male WAGR patient has undescended testes, surgery can be done to rectify it. In female WAGR patients it is important to have regular pelvic ultrasounds to check for gonadoblastoma.

Mental Retardation/Developmental Delays

Help for a WAGR patient with mental retardation can be received from early intervention services when he/she is born or diagnosed. Children with WAGR can also receive special education, physical therapy, speech therapy, and vision therapy.

Kidney Failure

WAGR patients should be regularly evaluated for high blood pressure and urinary proteins, which can be treated by medication. WAGR patients with renal failure usually also have high cholesterol, high blood pressure, and urinary protein. Some WAGR patients with renal failure can be treated with dialysis or a kidney transplant.

WAGR Study

A study of WAGR syndrome is being sponsored by the National Institute of Child Health and Human Development. For more information on this study or WAGR syndrome, please visit the International WAGR Syndrome Association website at http://www.wagr.org.

Gillespie's Syndrome

Gillespie's syndrome is a rare form of familial aniridia (autosomal recessive type), and accounts for 2% of aniridia patients. The classical triad of this syndrome is cerebellar ataxia (uncoordinated muscle movement from abnormality in the cerebellum), aniridia, and mental retardation.[20,21]

Cerebellar ataxia is a condition of poor muscle tone and difficulty in maintaining balance and coordination, which affects walking, writing, and speaking.

The severity of iris underdevelopment is less than in the typical aniridia patient. In addition to the aniridia, other eye findings include ptosis, nystagmus, and a small optic nerve. Patients with this syndrome do not develop cataract and corneal pannus.

Developmental delay, hearing deficiency, and pulmonic valve stenosis (blood cannot flow from heart to lungs sufficiently) have been reported in this syndrome. Fortunately, this syndrome is not associated with Wilms' tumor.[22]

Care should be taken to evaluate patients' physical and mental development in addition to their ocular development.

Associated Conditions

There are other conditions that are commonly found to be associated with aniridia.

Glucose Intolerance/Diabetes

As we know, the PAX6 gene is important in eye development. A recent study showed that the PAX6 gene is also involved in the development of endocrine cells in the pancreas.[23] Abnormalities in the PAX6 gene can cause impaired glucose-stimulated insulin secretion from the pancreas, which results in glucose intolerance and, in one report, diabetes mellitus.[24] Long-term diabetes mellitus unfortunately can be complicated by several medical and ophthalmologic problems such as cardiovascular compromise, diabetic retinopathy, and kidney failure. One should keep in mind that there is a high prevalence of glucose intolerance in patients with aniridia; therefore, glucose tolerance testing or regular blood glucose level should be included in the routine checkups.

Obesity

Obesity and intellectual disability occur in several genetic syndromes. It can be a reflection of lifestyle, unhealthy diets, and lack of exercise, but it has been reported as part of certain syndromes. Obesity and over-eating (hyperphagia) can be associated with WAGR syndrome.[25] The cause is unknown, but it is hypothesized that the gene for obesity could be located at the same chromosome as WAGR syndrome.[26]

Current research is showing that some patients with aniridia may also have issues with autism, glucose intolerance, and sensory disorder due to involvement of the PAX6 gene. For regularly updated information, please visit www.aniridia.net.

As mentioned, the PAX6 gene is responsible for the development of the eyes, but this gene can also affect the forebrain, kidneys, olfactory area, and pancreas. Each day there is new information and research being done on various conditions to see if they are linked with aniridia/WAGR. Some of these are:

- Glucose intolerance/diabetes—high blood sugar
- Autism—affects several parts of the brain, causing behavioral and cognitive problems such as speech and language delays; social isolation, hypersensitivity to sound, light, and textures; and insensitivity to potential dangers
- Sensory disorder—difficulty processing information from one's senses (sight, sounds, touch, taste, and smell)

Research is also being done on aniridia links to sleep disorders, auditory and verbal memory, and endocrine system problems. Each day more information is being found.

Other congenital anomalies that have been reported infrequently with aniridia/ WAGR syndrome are congenital heart defects, diaphragmatic hernia (weakening of the diaphragm resulting in the abdominal organ's moving into the thoracic cavity), tracheomalacia (under-development of the trachea), hearing deficiency, and absence of patella.[27]

In conclusion, aniridia, WAGR syndrome, and Gillespie's syndrome are conditions that can be associated with multiple systemic abnormalities. These need to be addressed early, including promotion of an understanding of the proper medical care needed to help patients lead a healthy life.

Notes

1. Gronskov, K., Olsen, J. H., et al. (2001). Population-based risk estimates of Wilms' tumor in sporadic aniridia: A comprehensive mutation screening procedure of PAX6 identifies 80% of mutations in aniridia. *Human Genetics 109*(1), 11–18.
2. Eagle, J., & Ralph, C. (2000). Congenital, developmental, and degenerative disorders of the iris and ciliary body. In Daniel M. Albert and Frederick A. Jakobiec (Eds.), *Principles and Practice of Ophthalmology*, 2 (pp. 1151–1153). Philadelphia: W.B. Saunders Company.
3. National Human Genome Research Institute (2009). Learning About WAGR Syndrome. January 29. Available at http://www.genome.gov/26023527
4. National Human Genome Research Institute (2009).

5. Jastaneiah, S., & Al-Rajhi, A. A. (2005). Association of aniridia and dry eyes. *Ophthalmology, 112*(9), 1535–1540.
6. Eagle (2000), 1151–1153.
7. Brandt, J. D., & Casuso, L. A., et al. (2004). Markedly increased central corneal thickness: An unrecognized finding in congenital aniridia. *American Journal of Ophthalmology, 137*(2), 348–350.
8. Mandal, A. K., & Netland, P. A., (2005). Secondary congenital glaucoma. In A. K. Mandal, P. A. Netland, & B. Heinemann (Eds.), *The Pediatric Glaucomas* (pp. 47–49). Amsterdam: Elsevier Butterworth Heinemann.
9. Nelson, L. B., Spaeth, G. L., et al. (1984). Aniridia. A review. *Survey of Ophthalmology, 28*(6), 621–642.
10. Nelson (1984), 621–642.
11. Eagle (2000), 1151–1153.
12. Nelson (1984), 621–642.
13. Nelson (1984), 621–642.
14. Eagle (2000), 1151–1153.
15. Day, S. (1997). Photophobia. In D. Taylor (Ed.), *Pediatric Ophthalmology* (pp. 1034–1036). Massachusetts: Blackwell Science, Inc.
16. Wammanda, R. D., & Idris, H. W. (2005). Aniridia associated with ptosis in three generations of the same family. *Annals of Tropical Pediatrics, 25*, 59.
17. National Human Genome Research Institute (2009).
18. National Human Genome Research Institute (2009).
19. National Human Genome Research Institute (2009).
20. Nelson (1984), 621–642.
21. Eagle (2000), 1151–1153.
22. Eagle (2000), 1151–1153.
23. Nishi, M., Sasahara, M., et al. (2005). A case of novel de novo paired box gene 6 (PAX6) mutation with early-onset diabetes mellitus and aniridia. *Diabetic Medicine, 22*, 641–644.
24. Yasuda, T., Kajimoto, Y., et al. (2002). PAX6 mutation as a genetic factor common to aniridia and glucose intolerance. *Diabetes, 51*, 224–230.
25. Amor, D. J. (2002). Morbid obesity and hyperphagia in the WAGR syndrome. *Clinical Dysmorphology, 11*(1), 73–74.
26. Tiberio, G., Digilio, M. C., et al. (2000). "Obesity and WAGR syndrome." *Clinical Dysmorphology, 9*(1), 63–64.
27. Clericuzio, C. L. (2005). WAGR Syndrome. In S. B. Cassidy and J. E. Allanson (Eds.), *Management of Genetic Syndromes* (pp. 645–651). Santa Fe, NM: Wiley-Liss, Inc.

2

Inspirations

JESSICA J. OTIS

This chapter is a collection of stories from those who do not let anything keep them from achieving their goals and who inspire us. These individuals show us there is hope and that anything is possible.

ERIC, USA—DON'T LET ANYTHING STOP YOU

My name is Eric, and I am 27 years old. I was born with familial (hereditary) aniridia. I also have nystagmus, beginnings of a cataract in my right eye, lens implant in my left eye, and corneal keratopathy in both eyes (but it is worse in my left eye). I am married to my lovely wife, Amber, and we have four children. They are: Joseph (ten years old), Sarah (seven years old), Aniston (four years old), and Christopher (two years old). The two oldest have normal vision and the two youngest have aniridia (how's that for the law of randomization?).

Currently, I work as a research assistant at the University of Florida as part of my doctoral degree. I also own my own company where I work as an occupational therapist with blind and low-vision individuals of all ages. Initially when I went to occupational therapy school, I was not interested in working with people who have vision impairments. Instead, I specialized in working with older adults. After working in the field for several years with older adults, I began to notice that many of my elderly patients had vision problems. Although I grew up with a visual impairment, I did not feel professionally qualified to address their vision issues because learning how to adapt to a visual impairment is different for someone born with a visual impairment than someone who acquires a visual impairment later in life. So I went back to school to gain additional training in working with people who have visual impairments. Part of my job as an occupational therapist is to evaluate patients for specific assistive-technology needs, recommend products that would increase their independence, and to teach patients with multiple disabilities how to use these devices. This experience has led to my interest in learning how to evaluate and train people with visual impairments in the use of assistive technology while at Florida State University FSU. Recently, I have used my new knowledge from FSU and my experience as an occupational therapist to create a company called Blind and Low Vision Rehabilitation Services & Consulting, Inc. Here I will be able to combine and utilize my personal and professional experience along with my academic knowledge to benefit the lives of people who have visual difficulties similar to mine. I have enjoyed this field tremendously and feel I can give a perspective regarding living with visual impairments that most professionals cannot give. I look forward to a long and rewarding career in this field.

Like many, I encountered roadblocks on my path to achieving this career, but many were dealt with early on while I was in elementary, middle, and high school. I attribute a lot of my success to my parents and to teachers of the visually impaired who helped me prepare for the many roadblocks I would face later in life. Not everything has been perfect in my pursuit. I have dealt with my fair share of prejudice from teachers/professors, employers, peers, and colleagues, but I was able to overcome this by having my mind set on a goal and letting no one deter me from achieving my goal.

If you are a parent reading this, the one thing I want to stress to you is to not to put limitations on your child with aniridia. Don't tell him/her what he/she can or cannot do. Don't tell him/her that one activity would be harder than another activity. Don't tell him/her that he/she should do one activity rather than another because of his/her eye condition. Instead, encourage your child's independence to try everything he/she can. Yes, at times your child might get hurt, but it is worse not to let him/her explore the limits of his/her own potential. In short, let a person with aniridia decide what his/her personal limits are, instead of defining his/he limits for him/her. If you do this then he/she might end up achieving more than you could ever imagine.

MATTHEW, USA—HAVING A VOICE

My name is Matthew, and I'm sixteen years old. I have sporadic aniridia, nystagmus, glaucoma, and a cataract. My mother and grandmother gave me the foundation upon which to challenge and fight the endless social injustices a blind person confronts, so, unlike many blind individuals, I was raised to be proud of my difference that made me part of a minority of people around the globe. I never had the shame that makes one vulnerable to bullying or teasing. However, if I had ever encountered this I would have explained my circumstance by trying to place the student in my shoes.

In school, my aide has strengthened my arguments for fairness by playing "devil's advocate" and has advised me on how to deal with the unfairness of the system until I am in a position to make a change. I was raised with the belief, not that I was equal to those who are sighted, but that I must be treated fairly and be given equal opportunities like everyone else. When I applied this philosophy to school, I encountered many injustices that can only be considered crimes committed by the system. These range from being denied Braille until third grade to being delayed or denied access to critical equipment that I needed. In spite of these obstacles, which prevent the success of thousands of blind individuals, I have maintained an A average throughout my entire schooling to date, and was recently admitted to the National Honor Society. While it is very easy for me to identify the numerous inaccuracies and failures of the system that slant the odds against my success, I do not believe isolation is the answer. If anything, integration to teach the sighted world about the difficulties and needs of those who are blind is the most important aspect of my schooling.

I believe the most difficult experience a blind person can have is trying to explain his/her circumstance to sighted individuals. For example, in math class, when fellow students were debating what game to play, such as hangman, on a half -day of school, it took my math teacher to remind the other students to be understanding, respectful, and inclusive. On a much broader topic, when my case manager tells me the cane is essential, I tell her to walk in my shoes blindfolded and put her life in the trust of a plastic stick.

My advice to all parents is that it is essential for their success and the success of future generations that people with aniridia stand up to the system that has unfortunately insured for the most part their failure for much too long. One way to begin and to give yourself and your child a voice is to join Aniridia Foundation International. AFI is very important and encouraging. Without such an organization, the minority of people with aniridia struggling to succeed would truly have no voice and would be left completely in the dark.

One thing I have done to advocate for the blind and visually impaired is that I recently wrote the U.S. Treasury Department. I wrote from a blind person's perspective. The following is what I wrote to them.

America is often associated with the ideals of freedom, liberty, and justice. From the perspective of a physically unique individual, America is more closely related to oppression of the minority, predetermined restrictions, and discrimination. My resentment is not of America or its principles, but of the social standards and expectations that make the American dream a remote possibility for people with differences.

While I am proud to be an American, I am not proud to be classified as a "blind individual." My visual ability to see the world in front of me may be compromised, but my ability to see social injustices is filled with clarity. I was raised in an environment based upon the entitlement to equal opportunity; however, this is not the reality of the life of a "blind man" in America.

Thousands of blind individuals across this nation accept the available and expected social modifications such as in mobility and in accessing information from the computer, without demanding better alternatives. Although these options involve suffering, struggling, and often failing, an impression of satisfaction, of not needing assistance, is given to the sighted world. In spite of their efforts, their worth is hardly recognized and acceptance is very slight. The sighted majority can only be granted an opportunity to understand and respect the difficulties of a blind person by being exposed to their differences. Only those who are ashamed of their uniqueness desire to conceal it with attempts towards independence for equality. I refuse to resign myself to the dismal hopes and bleak futures for blind people due to the odds stacked against their success.

The rules of the road that constrict 70% of blind people to a predetermined course of unacknowledged existence will not be the rules of my life. I perceive myself not as a disabled individual only deserving of minimum social modifications in order to be treated equally, but rather, as a unique individual entitled to easier access to achievable goals by being treated fairly. Independent skills are only part of the solution to compensate for the rougher road of someone in my situation. An independent voice that challenges injustices and refuses to settle for available, but insufficient options is the other key component.

I am this independent voice as I am neither sighted nor a visually challenged individual who blindly complies with society. While I do not fit either classification, my motives and actions are prompted, in the interest of all, for a more homogeneous existence. The blind should travel down their own side, independently and separately, all the while being understood better by sighted individuals. In this present situation, the sighted majority has the paved maintained side, while the blind minority has the neglected, broken asphalt side. The driving force behind this social contrast is the unrelenting sighted majority's persistent assimilation attempts. It must be recognized, and I will proudly admit it, that blind people have limitations in certain areas of life. This shall not be interpreted though to limit the freedoms and to mark off the aspirations of blind people. I am seeking to establish a standard of fairness under which the sighted world is adapted to the needs of the blind. Only under this standard can this severely biased road be evened to make "Liberty and Justice for All" a reality.

Based upon the beliefs and world perspective I have expressed, I would like to raise the issue of the unfairness of our currency. Sighted individuals take it for granted that they simply need to look with their eyes at a bill or coin to determine its value. Due to the absence of any tactile marks, a blind individual is reduced to having to scrape the edge of a coin and to estimate its weight in order to determine its value. Even more significantly, a blind person must trust a sighted individual in the transfer of bills; thus, creating the enormous vulnerability and defenseless of a blind person to being robbed. As an American my constitutional rights to property are being violated by the current denial for me to look with my fingers at the value of this nation's currency. Although this deprivation of rights is among many that blind people deal with as part of their oppressed existence, I cannot accept something that is unfair and unjust simply because it is the only thing available.

I am inquiring about the considerations and plans for the concerns I have addressed in terms of the currency. Specifically, what kinds of tactile marks are being considered? When is it planned for this adapted currency to be produced and to enter circulation? This matter should not be an issue of if, or how, unless the federal government has become so detached from the average citizen that it has forgotten its promise of being "of the people, for the people, and by the people." If light is not brought upon this issue as well as many others, blind people will still truly be left in the dark.

A second thing I have done to advocate for the blind and visually impaired is to get more books in Braille for all subjects. They are very difficult to get, which is extremely frustrating to me, to say the least. Right now I am working on applications for college. I am a senior in high school, treasurer of the student council, and a member of the National Honor Society. I am planning a career as a lawyer and advocate for people with disabilities so others won't have to fight to secure an equal education in public school and college. I intend to spend my life fighting for the rights of blind people and those with other disabilities to ensure equal access is guaranteed in every situation, including colleges, where special help is still rare. As a grandson of longtime activist Sylvia Guberman, I may be following her example. I already know it takes being aggressive to get things done. She has taught me that to make change, you have to work at it.

TRISCHA, USA—REACH FOR YOUR DREAMS

I was born with sporadic aniridia and slight nystagmus. I've had cataracts removed, and then three years ago had iris implants put in. For me the iris implants are wonderful for helping with glare. To anyone who is interested in iris implants I would say, first contact Price Vision Group in Indianapolis. I had my surgeries performed there, and my doctor was a true medical miracle worker for me and so many other people. Furthermore, if you do not take the risk of inquiring about the artificial iris implants, you will never know how your life could have changed. After I received the implants I went through bioptic training to learn to drive.[*] Today I feel more independent than ever thanks to being able to drive. After teaching for ten years I decided to make a career change. I had always been interested in law, so I attended law school. My current job right now is being a law clerk in the superior courts. The main emphasis is on civil cases. After clerking I would like to either pursue a litigation career or do something in copyright/trademark law. I chose these areas because I like the courtroom environment and I feel my sports background has produced the interest in copyright/trademark issues. I've never really found many roadblocks in trying to achieve my goals. The only thing that has tended to be a bit of a roadblock is people's overall perception of me until they get to know me. Once they get to know me, they have even more respect for me. For attorneys, many of the resources are on the computer, so I can use a magnifying program while using the computer. Throughout my life, my family and friends have given me the inward strength and drive to be successful. They were there to cheer me on when I won the Olympic gold medal in swimming. I always try to promote the availability and opportunities to individuals with aniridia, whether it is through encouragement or support. Being able to share my story with others through public speaking has been an ongoing goal. For my professional career I would like to be a positive and motivating practitioner within

---

[*] Editor's note: Please understand that any mention of the use of bioptic monocular glasses for driving does NOT mean that all people with aniridia are candidates to use these devices to drive. Nor do all states allow bioptic glasses for driving.

the legal community. So my one piece of advice for parents is to just let your child experience things a "normal" child would experience. Don't tell your child he/she can't do anything. Let your child adapt to do things, and the child will feel he/she is able to do things with his/her peers.

DOUG, USA—ADVOCACY FOR THOSE WITH DISABILITIES

I want to start by telling you what I have done during my life. I was born in 1953 in Schenectady, New York. My family moved to Utica, New York, around 1959, where I entered elementary school. My grandmother, father, sister, and I all have visual impairments. My sister and I did not have a diagnosis of aniridia until mid-life. We now believe that our deceased father and grandmother had aniridia. My vision history includes being in sight-saving class, near-vision being my best vision, not being able to see well enough to drive, and over time my vision getting worse. The doctors would say, "We can describe your vision loss, but don't have a name for it." The reason they were having difficulty was that I had an iris. A few short years later, my cornea pannus was taking most of my usable vision. I decided to go to college in Minnesota, where my parents are originally from, and this allowed me to be referred to see Dr. Edward Holland when he was in Minnesota. Dr. Holland did stem cell transplant, cornea transplants, and cataract surgery on my left eye, which returned my vision to 20/100. I am very happy with this result. Another doctor did the surgery in my right eye, but I experienced rejection in that eye. During this time I became familiar with AFI and currently I am an active volunteer with AFI. Then on March 8, 2006, I had KLAL surgery in my right eye. The recovery seemed normal enough. Dr. Holland did the surgery at St. Elizabeth's Surgical Center. A local doctor who had an internship and a fellowship at the University of Minnesota's Eye Clinic worked under Dr. Holland, and was involved with my surgery on my left eye and followed my progress.

While going to college I had an opportunity to have a roommate named Alan. Alan had a condition called Fredericks ataxia. This left him in an electric wheelchair and he needed assistance in his personal care. Alan was the first person to live on campus at Augsburg College who used an electric wheelchair for mobility. A new wheelchair-accessible dorm was built, and this is why Alan was able to live on campus. I was Alan's roommate that first year. During his second year in campus housing, I became his personal care attendant in addition to his roommate. Although the dorm was accessible, the rest of the campus was full of barriers, physical and otherwise. On a daily basis we confronted basic barriers to Alan's living and going to school. Many of the buildings were not wheelchair-accessible, and curb cuts did not exist. I remember pulling a manual wheelchair with Alan in it up stairs in two- and three-story buildings so that he could get up and down stairs to class and other activities.

I was the one that Alan came to and talked to about his many frustrations of being in a body that did not work well. I remember how people would hurt him. Some would not get his okay before pushing him to the college chapel, and others laid their hands on him and prayed that he would walk the next day and he became hopeful that he would be able to walk again. It was very painful for me to see him realizing he wasn't going to walk again. I also remember Alan going out into the community and talking to a manager of an apartment complex who said he would hire Alan, but the manager never called him. The manager did not return Alan's phone calls. Finally, Alan reached the manager and the manager said that he wanted Alan to leave him alone and that he never intended to hire him. These experiences hurt Alan, but somehow he would come around in a day or two and be positive about the future.

Alan's parents lived in upstate New York, and it so happened that his parents lived about seventy miles south of mine. I took him to my home to be with my family for a while over the Christmas break. Then I took him to his parents for a few days. Alan became my friend. He had not been home for fifteen years. Alan's disease caused his death in 1974 in a hospital room in the arms of his best woman friend from his church. I remember thinking I had a visual impairment and that it affected many things in my life, yet I felt that many others were faced with more barriers and life-threatening situations than mine.

I credit Alan as one of the starting places for my career and life of advocacy. Alan was one of the founding members of a Minnesota organization named the United Handicapper Federation (UHF). Part of my job was to take Alan to these meetings. I became a member and stayed involved. I became interested in a career in community-organized advocacy groups composed of people with disabilities, so in 1980 I started my master's program in rehabilitation counseling at Minnesota State University at Mankato. I have worked for the state Rehabilitation Services since 1992. During this time I have been a rehabilitation counselor, a placement specialist, a grant coordinator, and a specialist working in a grant-funded position. In my lifetime, I have seen people with disabilities becoming much more integrated into our society, and this makes me feel very happy. However, people with disabilities are still nagged by high unemployment rates that keep us from fully participating in the economics of our society. We must keep working on this and other issues.

Through a long personal process, I got the Minnesota State Service for the Blind to look at how it was treating its visually impaired and blind employees. Other visually impaired and blind employees did not jump onboard to support the idea right away, but privately told me, "Your ideas are good but we will never get it." Over many discussions with supervisors, co-workers, administration, and the department's Affirmative Action Officer, there were many give-and-takes about my reasonable-accommodation request. Then we started implementing my request for a paid driver and a state car. State Services for the Blind decided that if they were going to make this accommodation for me, they should give it to the other visually impaired employees. Every suggestion offered by administration was looked at as a way to control the employee. So the State Services for the Blind Administration and the visually impaired and blind staff discussed many different ways that the accommodations could be implemented. The visually impaired and blind staff was concerned that if the administration or supervisors took control of the hiring and scheduling of readers and drivers, it would not be an ideal situation to meet their needs. The visually impaired and blind staff stood together on wanting to take the responsibility to choose who would best meet their individual needs for a reader and/or driver. In part, this was due to mistrust of administration and the belief that a visually impaired or blind person would know best what their needs were and which person(s) would meet their needs. As much as possible, the visually impaired staff wanted the resources to hire and schedule the reader and/or driver. It took a couple to years to fully get implemented and develop a sense of trust. I was asked to help rewrite the department's affirmative action policy. Since then I have not had to worry about reasonable accommodation. The state now has a state job classification called "Reader/Driver Reasonable Accommodation" position. Since then, wherever I work they know that Doug Johnson will stand up for his reasonable accommodations. I learned that one person can make a difference in a big way. Since then, I truly see myself as an advocate. I do not believe all individuals with aniridia need to be advocates, but to this day I continue to advocate for people to live a full life, believe in themselves, and get out into the community.

Finally, I want to let you know that I am an advocate for all people with a special interest in those with disabilities. I like to help others overcome barriers. I also crave your friendship and rejoice in your successes. Like everyone else's, my life has had a lot of ups and downs, but I have learned enough about myself to be comfortable with who I am. My visual impairment was one of many factors in propelling me into my career. I want you to remember that I am a family member, I am a friend, I like to read and go to movies, I love living where I have mass transit so I can go places, I occasionally watch sports, I work full time, I volunteer part time for AFI, and, by the way, I have aniridia and it is a part of me. However, it is usually no big deal.

3

Aniridia—Epidemiology and Genetics

ANIL K. MANDAL AND HARSHA B. L. RAO

Aniridia literally means "without iris." The iris is the part of the eye that gives color to the eye. But the term *aniridia* encompasses more than its literal meaning and includes abnormalities of almost all the structures of the eye, from the cornea up to the optic nerve and including the angle of the anterior chamber, the lens, and the fovea. This is why aniridia is often called a "panocular disease."

The cornea is normally an avascular (lacking blood vessels), transparent tissue on the front part of the eye. In individuals with aniridia, it becomes vascularised. A bunch of blood vessels grows over the cornea: this growth is called a *pannus*.

The angle of the anterior chamber is that part of the eye between the cornea and the iris that drains the fluid within the eye out of the eye and maintains the pressure within the eye at normal levels. Aniridia affects this part and hampers the fluid flow out of the eye, thereby increasing the pressure within the eye, leading to a condition called *glaucoma*.

The lens is a biconvex structure behind the iris that focuses light rays entering into the eye onto the retina, which converts these light signals into electric signals that are carried through the optic nerve to the brain. In aniridia there may be displacement of the lens from its normal position, which is called *subluxation* or dislocation, or the normally clear lens may turn opaque, which is called a *cataract*.

The fovea is the area of the retina that is responsible for clear vision. It may be underdeveloped; this is called *foveal hypoplasia* and affects vision. Similarly, the optic nerve that carries the visual sensations may also be underdeveloped, affecting vision.

Besides these anatomical abnormalities, functional problems in addition to decreased vision include *nystagmus* (involuntary wobbling movement of the eye), squinting, and intolerance to light (*photophobia*).

In this chapter we will discuss mainly the epidemiology (incidence and distribution of diseases) and genetic aspects of aniridia. In the genetics part we will be discussing inheritance patterns, the gene responsible for the disease, other conditions associated with aniridia, and genetic tests available to detect the disease.

EPIDEMIOLOGY OF ANIRIDIA

Aniridia is not a very common disease in the population. Prevalence of aniridia varies from region to region. It is reported to occur in one out of every 61,000 members of the population in the United States; in Denmark the incidence is one in 96,000. Aniridia occurs equally in males and females, and no racial predilection has been described.

GENETICS

Aniridia occurs due to a defect in the PAX6 gene (described in detail later) located on the short arm of chromosome 11. These chromosomes have two arms known as "p"' and "q"' arms; p arm is the shorter arm and q arm is the longer arm. Genes are small segments of the genetic material known as DNA (deoxyribonucleic acid) that generally codes for protein and thus regulates some important functions in the body.

Inheritance Patterns

Each individual has two copies of every gene. One copy is inherited from the mother and the other from the father. If in an individual one copy of a gene is normal and the other copy is abnormal, and that person is normal, then that gene is said to show *recessive inheritance*, which means one abnormal copy of the gene is not sufficient to cause the disease. If in an individual one copy of a gene is normal and the other copy is abnormal, and that person has the disease, then that gene is said to show *dominant inheritance*, which means one abnormal copy is sufficient to cause the disease. If the gene shows an autosomal (non-gender) dominant inheritance pattern, then there is a 50 percent chance that the baby is going to get the disease, while in case of autosomal recessive inheritance this chance factor is 25 percent.

In terms of inheritance, there are four basic types of aniridia:

- Familial aniridia (autosomal-dominant)—This is the most common type of aniridia. It is due to mutations in the PAX6 gene. Here each baby of the affected parent has a 50 percent risk of having the disease.
- Sporadic aniridia—This type of inheritance is the second-most-common type. Here both the parents are normal and do not' have any chromosomal defects. The affected child has a new change in the PAX6 gene that probably occurred before or soon after conception. The cause for this change in the gene is not known. In addition to having features similar to familial aniridia, sporadic aniridia children are at risk of developing a type of kidney tumor called Wilms' tumor. This is a malignant tumor that has the ability to spread to other organs of the body. Children of patients with sporadic aniridia have a 50 percent chance of inheriting the disease if the change in PAX6 gene has occurred in the germ cells also.
- WAGR syndrome—This is a rare type of sporadic aniridia that occurs when both the parents are normal and the disease is due to a new mutation.

It differs from the more common form of sporadic aniridia in that the mutation involving the PAX6 gene also involves some neighboring genes on the short arm of chromosome 11. In addition to the common features of aniridia, children with WAGR syndrome have a high risk for developing Wilms' tumor; other medical complications, such as genital abnormalities; and learning and behavior difficulties. Early diagnosis and regular monitoring by a team of specialists is very essential in these cases.

- Gillespie syndrome—This is an extremely rare type of aniridia, accounting for only 2 percent of the total cases. It is inherited in an autosomal recessive manner; neither of the parents has any external features of aniridia. Each child of these parents has a 25 percent chance of inheriting the disease. These cases have a typical appearance of the iris remnant, a scalloped margin. In addition to the ocular features, these children also have associated mental retardation and difficulty in movement due to muscular in-coordination. However, unlike other forms of aniridia, Gillespie syndrome does not appear to be caused by mutations in the PAX6 gene.[1]

SYNDROMES ASSOCIATED WITH ANIRIDIA

The two syndromes associated with aniridia are discussed in detail below.

WAGR Syndrome

This is an extremely rare condition; it has been estimated that there are only about 300 cases worldwide. WAGR is an acronym that stands for the main symptoms of the disorder: Wilms' tumor, Aniridia, Genito-urinary abnormalities or Gonadoblastoma, and mental Retardation. For more detailed information on WAGR syndrome please see chapter one.

There are many additional conditions that can be associated with WAGR syndrome, of which two have recently been identified. One is a particular type of kidney dysfunction called *chronic renal failure*. Children with WAGR have a 40 percent chance of developing chronic renal failure, usually in their teens. This condition can occur in children whether or not they have a history of Wilms' tumor. The progression of this condition can be slowed with medications, so early identification of this condition is crucial. The other recently noted condition is *pancreatitis*, inflammation of the pancreas, the abdominal organ that secretes a hormone called insulin. Pancreatitis may lead to deficient secretion of insulin, and hence diabetes. Again, awareness and good medical care are essential in diagnosing and managing these conditions early.

Genetics

Early studies arrived at the conclusion that 30 percent of affected individuals with a family history of aniridia develop Wilms' tumor within the first five years of life. Subsequent studies revealed that the risk might be lower.[2] It is now known that these individuals with WAGR syndrome have a contiguous gene deletion (missing a part of a gene) encompassing both the 11p13 area, which contains the PAX6 gene, and the nearby region of 11p13, which contains a gene called the *Wilms' tumor suppressor gene* or WT1 gene. Absence of one WT1 allele in the germline in these individuals leads to a high risk (approximately 45 percent) of Wilms' tumor occurring through somatic mutation. Two genetic tests are required to check for WAGR syndrome. One is called the "karyotype," which is a basic examination of the chromosomes. The second test is called a "FISH" probe. The FISH probe is a very detailed examination of the WAGR-related portion of chromosome 11. Both tests are conducted on a small sample of blood.

GILLESPIE SYNDROME

Gillespie syndrome was first identified in 1965, and since then there have been only 21 reported cases: nine sporadic cases (with no family history) and 12 familial cases that occurred in five families. Though it is believed to be recessively inherited, studies in the familial cases have found a varying degree of similar symptoms in other family members, which suggests that it might be dominantly inherited (that is, one parent is affected and passes it on to his/her child).

Clinical Features

The major clinical features of this syndrome are:

- Bilateral partial iris hypoplasia—This means that in both eyes a part of the iris is missing. This makes the person appear to have very large and non-responsive pupils. It has also been clinically described as underdevelopment of the pupillary zone of the iris.
- Foveal hypoplasia—In people with Gillespie syndrome, vision is usually low but functional vision is still maintained. They can see where they are going and read normal print, though they may hold books and other objects closer to their faces than the average person.
- Nystagmus—Movement of eyes back and forth, up and down or in circular motion, also known as "wobbly eyes."
- Ptosis—Droopy eyelids or sleepy look.
- Aniridia is often milder in people with Gillespie syndrome than in people with isolated aniridia. People with Gillespie syndrome do not develop cataracts or corneal pannus, which are common in people with isolated aniridia.
- Congenital non-progressive cerebellar ataxia—The cerebellum is that part of the brain that is responsible for maintaining muscle tone, balance, and coordination. It does not control consciousness, thought, or intelligence. *Ataxia* means no coordination for movement. Cerebellar ataxia is a condition in which the muscle tone is poor; this causes difficulties in maintaining balance and coordination. This affects the child's ability to

walk unaided, to speak clearly, and to write. This is believed to be due to an underdeveloped cerebellum. The child's intelligence is usually normal and the content of the speech is normal. This combination of conditions often causes delayed development of both mental and motor skills.

The symptoms of Gillespie Syndrome can vary dramatically between individuals; however, all reported cases have shown both bilateral partial aniridia and cerebellar ataxia.

Genetics

No mutation or change of the PAX6 gene has been found in a patient with Gillespie syndrome, which suggests that people with Gillespie syndrome have a similar condition with a different origin.

GENETIC AND DEVELOPMENTAL BASIS OF ANIRIDIA

First documented as a genetic disease over 150 years ago, aniridia has since become a model for autosomal-dominant genetic disorders due to the high penetrance of its mutant genes, the ease of diagnosis at birth, and a similar incidence in various populations. It was only recently, however, that the aniridia gene was mapped on the short arm of chromosome 11, and this gene was called the PAX6 gene, a regulator of development of the eyes and central nervous system. There is a PAX6 dosage effect in aniridia ranging from mild loss of visual acuity and cataracts to severe nervous system defects and complete absence of the eyes (anophthalmia). PAX6 gene is a master regulatory gene that regulates the differentiation of major organ systems in the body. This means that this gene stimulates the development of different organs. "PAX gene" means *paired box* genes. There are other PAX genes, which are important for the development of the nervous system.

The PAX6 gene shows dominant inheritance, meaning one abnormal copy of the gene is sufficient by itself to cause the disease. If both the copies are abnormal in a person, it leads to a severe form of the disease. This can be lethal at birth or with severe abnormalities including absent eyes, large ears, defects in the nose, an underdeveloped brain, and abnormalities in the skull bones.

The molecular mechanism behind the dominant inheritance of aniridia is haploinsufficiency, where due to mutation one copy of the gene is not functional while the other copy cannot produce sufficient protein by itself to perform its function. All cases of aniridia are genetic, caused by mutations that prevent PAX6 from functioning normally in a person.[3] In about 98 percent of aniridia cases, these mutations can be in the form of deletion of a part of the chromosome 11, which contains the PAX6 gene, or change in the components of the gene so that the function of the gene is stopped. In the Gillespie syndrome cases of aniridia in which the PAX6 gene is normal, the mutation occurs in a region next to the gene itself and affects the ability of the PAX6 gene to be turned on in the eye; thus, these mutations are not detectable by screening for PAX6 mutations in the gene itself.

FISH ANALYSIS

This is a new technique that can be used to detect the mutations in the region of chromosome that contains the PAX6 gene. This technique consists of using fluorescent DNA segments (called *probes*) to attach to their complementary region on PAX6 gene on chromosome 11. The following figure (3.1) shows the normal position of PAX6 gene on the short arm of chromosome 11.

The genetic probes can be prepared if the genetic structure of the chromosome in that region is known. Figure 3.1 shows the genetic structure of a chromosome, which is actually the arrangement of what are called *nucleotides* in that region of the chromosome. These nucleotides are nothing but compounds whose arrangement in specific pairs makes up the genetic information within the genes. Each chromosome contains two strands that are connected to each other due to bonding between complementary nucleotides. Complementary nucleotides are those that can bond with each other and form pairs.

In the FISH technique, the first step is to break the paired strands of chromosomes into single strands by breaking the bond between them. Then a fluorescent genetic probe, which is basically a complementary copy of a portion of one of the strands of chromosome 11, is made to attach to its complementary part. This gives rise to fluorescence in the part of chromosome that contains the PAX6 gene. When there has been a change in that part of the chromosome at this region, the fluorescent genetic probe does not attach to this region and fluorescence is not detected after the test is done.

There are other techniques to find changes in the chromosome. One of them is called *karyotype analysis*. The chromosomes, when stained in order to see them with a microscope, look like strings with light and dark "bands." A picture (an actual photograph from one cell) of all 46 chromosomes, in their pairs, is called a *karyotype* (see Figure 3.2). A normal female karyotype is written 46, XX, and a normal male karyotype is written 46, XY. This

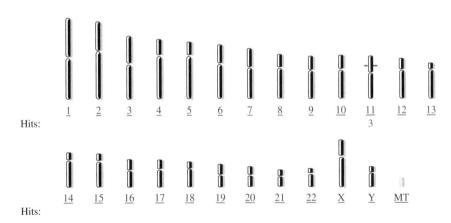

Figure 3.1 A color version of this figure may be viewed on the companion CD.

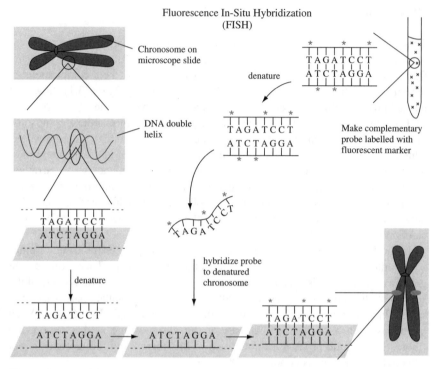

Figure 3.2 A color version of this figure may be viewed on the companion CD.

almost looks like the figure shown earlier of the chromosomes. The standard analysis of the chromosomal material evaluates both the number and structure of the chromosomes, with an accuracy of over 99.9 percent. Chromosome analyses are usually done from a blood sample (white blood cells), prenatal specimen, skin biopsy, or other tissue sample.

GENETIC COUNSELING

Genetic counseling provides individuals and families with information on the nature, inheritance, and implications of genetic disorders to help them make informed medical and personal decisions. The following section deals with genetic risk assessment and the use of family history and genetic testing to clarify genetic status for family members.

Isolated Aniridia and WAGR Syndrome

Isolated aniridia and WAGR syndrome are inherited in an autosomal-dominant manner. Risk to family members is based on the mode of inheritance.

Parents of an Isolated-Aniridia Child

The majority of individuals diagnosed with aniridia have an affected parent. A child with isolated aniridia may have the disorder as the result of a new change in the PAX6 gene called *de novo* gene mutation.[4] Because the severity of the condition may vary greatly among family members, both parents should be examined for evidence of minor degrees of iris hypoplasia or reduced visual acuity caused by foveal hypoplasia.

Siblings of a Child with Isolated Aniridia

The risk to the siblings of the affected child depends upon the genetic status of the child's parents. If a parent of the affected child has isolated aniridia or has an identifiable PAX6 mutation, the risk to the siblings is 50 percent. When the parents are clinically unaffected, the risk to the siblings of an affected child appears to be low.[5]

Offspring of an Affected Individual

Each offspring of an affected individual with isolated aniridia has a 50 percent chance of inheriting the PAX6 mutation and developing aniridia.[6]

Parents of a WAGR-Affected Child

WAGR syndrome caused by a gene deletion detected only by FISH testing or heterozygosity testing usually occurs *de novo*; however, rarely, an asymptomatic parent may have an deletion that does not manifest; thus, it is appropriate to offer FISH testing or heterozygosity testing to both parents. In individuals with WAGR caused by a cytogenetically visible deletion, it is appropriate to offer cytogenetic testing to both parents to determine if either has what is called a *balanced chromosome rearrangement*, because this condition increases the risk for other offspring.

Siblings of a WAGR-Affected Child

If a parent has a balanced chromosome rearrangement, the risk to the siblings is increased, depending on the nature of the chromosome rearrangement. If the affected child has a *de novo* contiguous gene deletion and neither parent has evidence of *mosaicism* (a condition where some cells are normal and some cells are abnormal, with changes in the structure or number of chromosomes) for the deletion, the risk to siblings is no greater than that in the general population.

Offspring of an Affected Child

Individuals with WAGR syndrome generally do not reproduce.

RELATED GENETIC COUNSELING ISSUES

Considerations in Families with an Apparent *De Novo* Mutation

When neither parent of an affected child with an autosomal-dominant condition has the disease-causing mutation or clinical evidence of the disorder, it is likely that the affected child has a *de novo* mutation. However, possible nonmedical explanations could also be explored, including alternate paternity or undisclosed adoption.

Family Planning

The optimal time for determination of genetic risk and discussion of the availability of prenatal testing is before pregnancy.

DNA Banking

DNA banking is the storage of DNA (typically extracted from white blood cells) for possible future use. Because it is likely that testing methodology and our understanding of genes, mutations, and diseases will improve in the future, consideration should be given to banking DNA of affected individuals. DNA banking is particularly relevant in situations in which the sensitivity of currently available testing is less than 100 percent.

Prenatal Testing

Prenatal testing using fetal cells obtained by amniocentesis usually performed at about 15–18 weeks' gestation, or chorionic villus sampling (CVS) at about 10–12 weeks' gestation, are available under the following circumstances:

- For pregnancies at increased risk for isolated aniridia if the disease-causing PAX6 mutation of an affected family member has been identified
- For pregnancies at increased risk for WAGR caused by a cytogenetic deletion if a balanced chromosome rearrangement has been identified in a parent
- For pregnancies at increased risk for WAGR caused by a cryptic deletion detectable by FISH or heterozygosity testing

Preimplantation Genetic Diagnosis (PGD)

Preimplantation genetic diagnosis may be available for families in which:

- The disease-causing PAX6 mutation has been identified in an affected family member in a research or clinical laboratory.

- A chromosome rearrangement detectable by chromosome analysis, FISH, or heterozygosity testing has been demonstrated in a parent.

Genetic counseling has also come a long way in predicting the chances of an offspring's getting affected. Until newer genetic therapies become available, genetic counseling will play a major role in reducing the incidence of the disease. However, studies regarding the inheritance and genetic aspects of aniridia have opened up new avenues into further research aimed at tackling the disease. In the future we may see new management strategies at the genetic level to modify the course of the disease or to prevent the inheritance of the disease.

Notes

1. Lauderdale, J. D., (2007). Personal communication, March 29.
2. Dome, J. S., & Huff, V. (2005). Wilms' Tumor Overview. Available at: http://www. geneclinics.org/servlet/access?id=8888890&key=lgVrnDkFEBGMk&gry=INSERTGRY&fcn=y&fw=4KHW&filename=/glossary/profiles/wilms-ov/index.html.
3. Lauderdale, J. D. (2007).
4. Dome, J. S., & Huff, V. (2005).
5. Dome, J. S., & Huff, V. (2005).
6. Dome, J. S., & Huff, V. (2005).

4

Personal Experiences of
Individuals with Aniridia

JESSICA J. OTIS

No one can make you feel inferior without your consent.

—Eleanor Roosevelt

Editor's Note: Since not much was known about aniridia for many years some doctors did medical procedures that we now know should not be done on aniridic eyes. Please do not use any specific story here as a guide for your journey, since some of the medical procedures mentioned should not have been done. Furthermore, please make sure to see a doctor with experience and knowledge of anirida. Lastly, please keep in mind, each person's journey has different medical issues. Not everybody will experience the exact same medical challenges in their journeys. Many people affected by aniridia go through similar experiences. Some deal with bullies differently than others, and some may have difference experiences with employment-related issues. Whatever experiences you have had in your life, these stories will show that you are not alone. Many others have felt and gone through situations similar to ones you have gone through. It is our hope that these stories inspire and help you with any struggles you may have now or in the future.

ACCOMPLISHMENTS

Mark, United States—You can do anything!

I was born with a case of sporadic aniridia in 1976 in Maui, Hawaii, to my parents, Mike and Pat. I have one brother two years older who has normal vision, but my mom had a miscarriage of a girl with the same aniridia condition.

I had a normal childhood, doing everything the majority of kids did, including soccer, Cub Scouts, body surfing, boogie boarding, and bicycling. In my early teens I competed in outriggered canoe racing. This was questioned due to my vision, but my six-man crew placed first in the state championship regatta. This experience inspired me to continue in the area of sports and enjoy them while testing my limits, which was done with cross-country running and track and field in high school.

When I graduated from Maui High School in 1994, it was considered a great accomplishment by my parents and many teachers who had doubts about my learning abilities due to the inability to read the work written on the board. My own efforts had to be supplemented with handwritten notes by other students or teachers to make up what I missed. After high school I went to the University of Northern Colorado. I graduated in 1998 with a degree in kinesiology, emphasizing exercise science and with a minor in dietetics. I continued my education and love of the human body in Colorado Springs at the Colorado Institute of Massage Therapy, and got my degree in massage therapy.

I lived in Colorado Springs for five years and worked various jobs, which tested my education, willpower, and mindset for equal treatment. I worked at the YMCA as a personal trainer for two years, and suffered the trials of discrimination by supervisors due to the physical appearance of my eyes. This experience was investigated by the Equal Employment Opportunity Commission, but was never brought to trial due to unusual missing evidence. My experiences also included working as a physical therapy assistant, a massage therapist and teaching at a newly opened massage school. My work experience in Colorado Springs culminated at a twenty-four-hour fitness facility as one of their specialized personal trainers who held three certifications. They were from the National Strength and Conditioning Association (NSCA), International Sports Science Institute (ISSI), and United States Olympic Weight Lifting (USAW). These certificates allowed me the opportunity to work with populations of athletes, patients undergoing rehabilitation, and those with special needs.

In addition to my work experience in the health and fitness world in Colorado Springs, I continued competing in sports to test my physical limits of body and vision. I competed regularly in road racing, triathlons, and adventure races. Fortunately, I did not have any accidents or injuries due to my vision impairment, but always kept a different mindset to keep trying no matter what anyone else may have thought. My athletic experiences in Colorado Springs did bring me good fun, and the luxury of sponsorship by two local running shoe stores who paid for equipment and races for me.

The final part of my story brings me to my current life in Hayward, California. I made the decision to come to California for my greatest challenge: to prove to myself that I am enabled, not disabled. I came to California and started my final schooling for a chiropractic doctorate at Life West Chiropractic College. This is a field that is testing my full mental and visual ability, which can be described as totally challenging, honorable, and humbling. I am in quarter five out of fourteen of the program, and have already hit huge hurdles of testing trials and tribulations. I am supported by many of the faculty and students, and despised by others who doubt me just for my lack of vision. The study load is equal to that of any medical school program and can be overwhelming at times, with insufficient amounts of sleep and mindless relaxation. The finishing of the program is in sight; even though it is two and half years away, my passion for and enjoyment of it grow each day, making the challenge all the more worth it. There have not been many blind chiropractors graduating from such programs. One did so thirty years ago, and another recently finished who is blind as a result of diabetes. My goal is to finish this degree and start a successful wellness clinic of chiropractic in which I will be able to help many to learn how to improve the quality of their lives, as many have done for me.

Janet, United States—Accomplishments Take Time and Hard Work

When I attended the Aniridia Foundation International's 2005 medical conference in Chicago, I was amazed at the services that are available today, which did not exist forty-five years ago.

Today, an obstetrician has to examine a baby for aniridia and, if it is found, must call in a pediatric ophthalmologist to check for cataracts and glaucoma. When my mother took me home from the hospital, she sat on the sofa next to a lamp with me in her arms. She looked at my face and realized she could see all the way to the back of my eyes. Because she had two other children, she knew something was wrong.

She found a doctor who knew it was aniridia, and that I was one in a million. I was born with aniridia, myopia, congenital cataracts, astigmatism, and nystagmus. He said the aniridia was caused by genetics or rubella. My parents "shook the family tree" and found nothing. My mother did not remember having rubella, and was told it could be a slight case with just a headache and no rash. Today, rubella has been discounted, and the genetic factor could come from fourteen generations ago.

I started wearing thick, dark, rose-colored glasses at the age of fourteen months. I hated them and tried to throw them away. As I grew, I heard the phrase "lens changes," but I never heard the word "cataract" until I was forty-two. I was tested for glaucoma as a teenager and put on pilocarpine. During my childhood and early adulthood, I was told that any eye surgery was impossible. Fortunately, the pilocarpine controlled the eye pressure.

I attended a sight-saving class for grade school and then went to a normal junior high school. Because my parents were concerned about sending me to a large high school, they sent me to a private girls' school where I was in a class of twenty. Following graduation, I attended a small liberal arts college and received my bachelor of arts degree four years later. During my childhood, my eyeglass prescription changed annually. By my senior year in college, my vision had stabilized so that I could wear contact lenses. They were black, hard lenses, which kept out the glare and improved my vision through glasses, especially by giving me full peripheral vision. Through these lenses, my vision was consistently 20/70 for eighteen years.

Following graduation, I tried to find a job, but I was hampered by my vision and my gender. Today, there is a joke, "You have a college degree. That's wonderful. Can you type?" Forty-five years ago it was not a joke, but reality. Because of my math background, I tried for an engineering assistant job. I filled out my own application, took a battery of timed tests and passed, and interviewed for the job. I then began the medical exam by reading the eye chart. Large manufacturing companies required at least 20/40 visual acuity.

In one company, I was told they would accept me for a clerical position with a substandard medical rating if I could pass the shorthand and typing tests. I didn't. At another company, the manager was ready to hire me, but I had to go to the medical department. When I flunked the eye chart, they used medical insurance as their excuse. As I left the medical department, I said to myself, "What do I have to do to get a job?" I broke down and sobbed.

Someone recommended that I go to the Association for the Blind. (Today, it is the Association for the Blind and Visually Impaired.) When the receptionist handed me the application, she asked if I needed help. I replied, "No, thank you." I filled out the form and returned it. She then exclaimed, "I'm sorry, we cannot help you. Your vision is too good." Her response made me one of thousands who "fell between the cracks."

A woman at my church was able to obtain a position for me in her company, where she had broken through the "glass ceiling." The medical exam consisted of a nurse's asking me questions, one of which was, "Can you see well enough to do the job?" and I answered in the affirmative. This was an insurance company. Over seven years, I received several promotions. During that time, I returned to school at night to learn about computers, and upon graduation I started a thirty-one-year career in information technology. My first position was in state government, which had no medical exam. Future jobs were always with the insurance industry or government. Today, discrimination is against the law.

I always worked as a normal person, with no request for special equipment. Because I do not drive a car, my job had to be in a location where I could use public transportation. Throughout this time, I was able to travel nationally and internationally, alone or in groups.

When I was forty, I was told that surgery was no longer impossible but still very tricky. After wearing my contacts for eighteen years, I was advised to buy a new pair because of the many scratches on my cornea. The new pair was too tight, though, and allowed blood vessels to grow on the cornea. The doctor took a wait-and-see attitude. When I changed doctors, I was told to stop wearing them, but it was too late; the damage was permanent. The corneas also suffered scar tissue. My first surgery was at age forty-six to scrape off the scar tissue from the right cornea.

One doctor, who had only a textbook knowledge of aniridia, told me to use Timoptic™ instead of pilocarpine. My pressure, which had been controlled for over twenty years, increased. When I asked to be put back on pilocarpine, he responded that pilo works on the iris and, since I do not have an iris, it cannot work. As he increased the Timoptic, the pressure increased. He finally allowed me to use the pilocarpine in addition to the Timoptic. The right eye pressure was restored, but the left eye required filter surgery at age forty-eight. Later, I was told that because my iris can be seen under a microscope there is sufficient iris for pilocarpine to work.

My cataracts were first detected at age forty-two, back when lenses were removed and people wore thick glasses. Because eye surgery was still "tricky" for aniridia patients, my surgery was delayed for nine and ten years, when the lenses were replaced with lens implants. Then further right corneal scarring was scraped by an excimer laser, and I continued to have glaucoma problems. Both eyes required surgery to implant the Ahmed[TM] Glaucoma Valve.

Twice I was sent to a corneal specialist for a possible corneal transplant, but was turned down because the aniridia might reject the new cornea. After September 11th, 2001, my sister in Cincinnati saw a news item about aniridia and called me with the information. I made an appointment and saw Dr. Edward Holland before Christmas when my left eye vision was 20/400. The right eye only had a sliver of peripheral vision. Even though he took pictures, he could not see the optic nerve, but the glaucoma doctor felt it was worthwhile doing the right eye. Only after stem cell and corneal transplants were done could he see that the optic nerve was 95 percent damaged. The steroids for the surgeries continued increasing eye pressure. The only solution was Diamox, which I am able to tolerate.

Once the right eye was complete, stem cell and corneal transplants were done on the left eye, giving me 20/125, which then became 20/160. The left optic nerve is 70 percent damaged. I was weaned off the oral immune suppression drugs. Because of the immune suppression eyedrops, any scratches on the cornea can lead to ulcers. An ulcer on each eye after Thanksgiving of 2005 required strong toxins to kill the bugs, but they also affected the stem cells. By using the oral immune-suppression drugs, we enabled the stem cells to become viable again, but the ulcers had left scar tissue, which required a corneal transplant of the left eye. After I lived through more than three months of being blind, the transplant was performed on Monday, and I did my income taxes on Friday. My left vision was restored to 20/160. As the sutures were removed, the stem cells continued to improve. In spite of the struggles, it has been a wonderful life.

Roger, United States—Accomplishments in Career

I was born with familial aniridia. I live in Fredericktown, Missouri, with my wonderful wife, Wendy, and our four smart, talented children (of course, I'm not biased in any way).

My experiences in school were pretty good. The Americans with Disabilities Act (ADA) and the Individuals with Disabilities Education Act (IDEA) were not in effect during the time I was in school, but the teachers seemed to work well with the accommodations I needed. If I had a barrier, I would work with the teacher, the office, and my VI (vision impairment) teacher, and we would find a solution.

After graduating from high school, I attended Southeast Illinois College for about a year. I moved from southern Illinois to southern Indiana, and began taking part-time classes at Ivy Tech College in Evansville while working full time in a factory. I was studying computer programming at Ivy Tech when a problem arose. A main portion of the coursework depended on accessing bits of information within a mainframe computer system. The rest of my work was accessible, but the technicians could not download the magnification software. So, out of frustration, I gave up that endeavor.

Since that time, I've tried many things. In the process, I have received a certificate in business and an associate of arts degree in education. Due to having multiple complications associated with aniridia, it has been challenging for me to acquire technology that can help me reach my dreams. Many times, I have accomplished short-term goals only to find out that the long–term goal was unrealistic due to a lack of usable technology.

In 2000, I attended Partners in Policymaking. In this nine-month training, I learned how to advocate more effectively for change. It focused on many things, including advocating for legislative changes or simply a better IEP (Individualized Education Program) for your child. Since then, I've joined multiple boards and participated in many activities to advocate for change. Currently, I am working through an Americorps VISTA project called Missouri Community Advocates Network (MoCAN). One of the key purposes of this project is to promote a change in perceptions that will impact how all people with disabilities are included in their community. By focusing on people as a whole, we strive to eliminate the myths of differences. A person with aniridia is no different from a person who is "normal"; and by the same token, that person is no different from a person with autism or a cognitive disability. We demonstrate these opinions through interactive presentations.

I plan to start school in the fall to complete my bachelor's in special education, and I hope to get my certification to become a VI teacher. My hope is to help youths who are transitioning to set goals, which will maximize their potential and utilize all of the technology available. My experiences have given me a wealth of knowledge to draw from in many things, and this should be an asset for students when looking at alternatives.

Mike, United States—Struggles and Successes

Joy, happiness, and excitement are some of the emotions experienced by parents and their families on the birth of a child. These emotions can be dampened by the news that their child has a disability. I was born with aniridia, and I'd like to share some of my struggles and successes with you. I believe that having a visual disability is one of the hardest disabilities to overcome.

I was born on March 28, 1989, to Jill Nerby. She was the second person in the state of Wisconsin to be diagnosed with aniridia in the winter of 1961–1962. Thus, I have familial aniridia. When I was about twelve, I developed glaucoma. I have had nystagmus since birth (shaking eyes), but it is only noticeable when I am tired. My corrected vision (with glasses) in my right eye was last measured at 20/70 and my left was 20/200. I was lucky to have enough vision to function somewhat normally.

One of the first problems that I noticed was light glare because I don't have an iris. (This is the colored part of your eye. It controls how much light is let into your eye.) I squint, and some say my eyelids droop. As a kid I would have people think I was on drugs. Other kids would say things like, "Man, you are stoned! Can I get some of that stuff you're smoking?" or "Dude, look, that kid is blazed out of his mind." Also, just my eyes looking different was a basis for kids to make fun of me by saying things like, "Hey, Mike, how many fingers am I holding up?" or "Hey, Stevie Wonder." You have to believe in yourself so the insults will not emotionally overtake you. You need to understand that there are people in life who are ignorant and mean, and you do not need to be like them. I would just ignore them and eventually the bullying would stop. If it didn't, then I was forced to stand up for myself and confront them about what they were saying about me. Although I do not advocate physical violence, if need be, defend yourself (but do not initiate conflict). I found that people respected me more for standing up to the bullies.

Next, I struggled with the many surgeries that many people with aniridia need to keep their vision. I was in high school while I was having the glaucoma surgeries and stem cell transplants. In addition, about three times I was scheduled for a transplant and it was cancelled due to lack of tissue. This was emotionally like being on a roller coaster. Getting your hopes up, having fears, getting your nerves worked up to go through it; then you're let down and get disappointed. But you still have the fear until the surgery is rescheduled; then the hopes then rise again, and it is a vicious emotional circle. There is also stress from missing schoolwork. However, no matter the downside, surgery was very much worth it.

As I have grown and have begun to try to find a job, I have found that employers don't want to hire me due to the way my eyes look. They won't admit that is the reason why, but I can tell that's why. A good example would be at a certain restaurant. Since I was thirteen I worked during the summers at a different restaurant in Wisconsin. We knew the owner and he agreed to give me a job. I was raised to believe that if I wanted something I had to work for it, and in Wisconsin you can work beginning at thirteen. When I was twelve I went up to the man and said, "Sir, next summer I will be thirteen. If I come up here (Wisconsin) for the summer, can I work for you?" He later told my mom, "Any kid that wants to work at thirteen has to be a hard worker," and he wanted hard workers working for him. When I was sixteen, knowing I had experience from working during the summers at that restaurant, I applied at another in the fall to earn a little extra money. I didn't care if I had to start at the bottom. They turned me down, saying that in Tennessee you couldn't have a minor working after ten o'clock on a school night, and they closed at ten. I was thinking, alright, no big deal. When I was nineteen, having accumulated five years of restaurant experience, I applied at this restaurant again. I wanted to be a waiter or cook, having experience as both, but I was open to any job they had available. They called me back for an interview. The interview was on a Wednesday afternoon and it went great. I told him about aniridia and my vision, and he seemed somewhat concerned about my vision if he were to hire me as a waiter. I quickly attempted to put his mind at ease, reassuring him that my vision was good enough that I could do the job as well as someone who had perfect vision. The manager said, "We'll call you back for a second interview in a couple days." Knowing that I was no longer a minor and had experience, I thought that this was a good sign that I would get the job. Friday rolled around and I didn't get a call from them. I thought, no big deal, it is Friday, maybe the guy took the day off or something. On Monday I called and the manager informed me that they had hired everyone they needed on Friday.

As far as jobs are concerned, I'm not quite sure what the best approach is yet, but personally, I tell them up front so they can't fire me and say that I was withholding information about myself. I have found no difference in the success rate of my being employed if I tell them up front or if I don't tell them at all about my vision.

In addition, I have encountered uninformed teachers, which has posed a great threat to me academically and athletically. As part of my Individual Education Program (IEP), I was allowed to wear a hat in school to help reduce the amount of glare from the florescent lights. In sixth grade, one of my teachers told me to take off the hat. I tried to explain the situation to her. I guess she thought I was making stuff up. Like I would make up being legally blind just to wear a hat in school. She then pushed me against a locker and forcefully removed my hat. Another example of uninformed teachers occurred when I was in eighth grade. I wanted to play football, and the head coach asked my mom, "If I put Mike on the line, can he see the guy in front of him?" This seemed funny to me, especially after I had sought him out by myself and introduced myself to him. I was on the team for about a month. After going to all the practices and running the drills as well as most of the kids with better vision, I had gotten very little if any playing time when we would have a scrimmage during practice. I got the sense that the coach was afraid to play me, thinking I might get hurt. I quit the team and have regretted that decision ever since. I feel that I should have stuck with it no matter what the cost to prove to him that I wouldn't have gotten injured due to being visually impaired.

Athletics are very important to me, and I love being involved with them no matter what role I play. During the spring of my freshman year in high school, I approached the football team's defensive coordinator (who just so happened to be my gym teacher that year). I asked him if there was any way that I could assist the football team. He sent me to talk to the head coach He let me be a manager and assisted me in finding a summer camp for high school students who wanted to be athletic trainers. Starting in the fall of my sophomore year, my role was manager/trainer; over time it morphed into whatever needed to be done, culminating in my senior year when I shot, edited, and produced the varsity football and baseball teams' highlight DVDs. My senior year, another coach joined our coaching staff. Over the course of the season I became closer to him, and he is one of the two coaches who I look up to as mentors and who have inspired me to want to become a teacher and coach. The other coach was the defensive coordinator, and he helped me with writing letters for scholarships and got me a position on Western Kentucky University's football team as a manager.

In my senior year I picked up bowling for the first time in six or seven years and became a starter for the varsity bowling team. Around late September, after questions had been raised about the boys' team captain's commitment, several of the boys' and girls' team members came to me. They said that I should be named team captain, and even if I wasn't they still would look at me as the team captain. This was an unbelievably powerful message to me, since I had joined the team a month before. I have stuck with bowling and most recently bowled scores of 213, 211, and 202. This year I finished in the top ten in the city, with my four-man team finishing second. The bowling coach was a great teacher, and he nominated me for a scholarship called *Beat the Odds* for teens who overcome large obstacles in their lives and succeed with excellence. I was very proud to win it, but even prouder to know that people looked at me with pride for my attitude and accomplishments, not pity.

After I had gotten settled in with football and bowling, in October of my senior year I joined the prom committee. I received an incredible compliment from the principal. He picked me out of a student body of 2,500-plus to be chairman of finance. A teacher later told me, "He picked you because he knew that you were trustworthy and responsible enough to take on such an important position." It was a great experience, but nerve-wracking at the same time because I had to make decisions on food, decorations, etc., and then try to balance all of the spending because we had to leave a set amount in the account for the next year's prom.

In addition to academics, football, bowling, and prom committee, I was a three-year starter for my church basketball team. Over the course of three years I played every position. During my last year we finished with a 9–1 record.

In conclusion, teachers and the general public need to be more informed about disabilities, specifically visual disabilities. For example, some teachers think just putting you in the front row is enough to help. They do not understand someone with a visual impairment needs more than that. Also, public arenas, concert halls, or sporting facilities have special seating for the disabled, but in most places it is in the back of the room or away from the stage where wheelchairs have easy access. There is no up-close seating available for the visually impaired, unless you want to pay the higher prices of the close seating. Although, once some dedicated teachers understand your situation, most of them are more than willing to help you any way they can. My best advice for finding success is to find something that you enjoy and just work at it. You might have to work harder to get where normal-sighted people are, but in the end you are going to work hard at anything you want to do well. If you want it badly enough, you will work hard enough to attain your goals, and you will succeed.

ADVOCACY

Debbie, United States—You're not Alone

I'm 49 years old. I was diagnosed with aniridia at two years old. I am from and currently living in Fostoria, Ohio, which is a small community of about 14,000. I enjoy spending time in my flower gardens and taking care of them, and also making floral arrangements. I also enjoy baking cookies for my local low-vision support group, which is called As Eye See It. We meet once a month. I love to collect recipes, birds (artificial), and birdhouses. I also can't forget about my computer, which I enjoy very much and is how I found Aniridia Foundation International (AFI). I am so glad that I did.

I am a homemaker. I have sporadic aniridia. Other eye conditions I have are keratitis, cataracts, and nystagmus. My vision acuity is 20/400. I don't wear glasses now, but I used to until they really didn't help and I became legally blind. I wear prescription sunglasses most of the time to block out the bright lights and glare. Growing up for me wasn't that bad; I really didn't know anything different. I thought everyone saw things the same way as I did, but I didn't put too much importance on it at the time, since I could still see fairly well. Being from a small community and being the oldest of five children, I felt I needed to help others more than I needed help. I am the only one in my family with aniridia. I am thankful for my parents not stopping me from trying things and experiencing different obstacles of life: for example, going skating and bowling with friends. During college I got my degree in elementary education. I do not drive. I always had hope that someday I would be able to drive. I hoped that my eyes would get better or some discovery of something would help me see better. I did take the book part of driver's education in my sophomore year, which I did pass, but I couldn't do the driving part. I couldn't pass the eye exam. I walk to nearby places using my white cane, or my husband drives me to places I want or need to go. For the most part I think I'm independent. I always try to do things myself instead of having someone do it for me. I guess I like the challenge to see if I can accomplish the task. I feel comfortable telling other people when they are truly interested in my condition. It's usually people that have something in common with me and they understand what I am going through, because they have experienced the same thing or something similar.

I would be very sad and feel very alone without AFI. I was always told that aniridia was very rare and that I was the only person in my area with it, and doctors really didn't know that much about it, it was just an unfortunate thing that just happened. So I had to accept the fact and learn to live with it. I am sure glad that after all these years I know now that I'm not alone. Thank you, AFI, for all the support and information that you have given me. I feel like I won a million dollars! I like the fact that you can share ideas, information, or problems with others who are trying to cope with the same thing that you are, which is aniridia. So being a member is very important to me.

The most difficulty that I have experienced is when I took mobility lessons for using a white cane. The actual lessons weren't that difficult, it was acceptance of the fact that, to be independent, I needed to learn how to use the cane. Now I take it with me every time that I leave the house. I have several people who have helped and inspired me. My parents and my husband have inspired and supported me in good and bad times, and in achieving my goals.

Marilyn — Be Your Own Advocate

I was born with sporadic aniridia. I also have nystagmus, cataract, and corneal pannus. I have to wear contacts to help me see better, and with them my vision acuity is 20/80. Currently, I am waiting for a possible stem cell transplant for my corneas. Growing up I was very fortunate to have a wonderful support group of family and my eight close friends whom I grew up with and still keep in touch with. The one thing that was and still can be difficult for me is not being able to drive. It was frustrating and made me feel as though I was robbed of independence. But I got through it all because of my support group and because of having a positive attitude. I would think of Helen Keller and how she overcame even tougher struggles than mine. Many others have something worse than aniridia, and we must remember that to help us stay positive when we have challenges in our lives. We should not pity ourselves, because we need to be our own advocates.

Today I have three wonderful daughters who are all in college. While my girls were growing up, we used carpooling and my husband as modes of transportation until my daughters were old enough to drive. My youngest daughter, Rachel, has aniridia. When Rachel was first born, I was a little upset, then I became even more nervous after finding out about WAGR syndrome and testing for Wilms'. I had never heard of it before and was never tested for Wilms' tumor when I was a child. I felt bad for passing aniridia on to her because of my sense of responsibility for taking care of her. However, today Rachel is doing well in college in Indiana. She sometimes uses a monocular to see things. Also being assertive and not shy helps Rachel be her own advocate. I feel it is important for parents to make sure their children have a strong support group of family and friends. Allow your child to have a "normal" life and teach him/her to be his/her own advocate.

STRUGGLES

Rosemarie, United States—Struggles and Strain on Relationships

Living with aniridia has not always been easy and has permeated every aspect of my life. The biggest part of my life that has been affected is my relationship with my parents and sisters.

My relationship with my parents is kind of strange. We both feel guilty and like we need to compensate. My parents feel guilty; at least my dad does, because I inherited aniridia from him, and they never wanted any of their children endure it. They also feel guilty because I will never be able to live up to what I really want to be, since there will always be limits because of my vision. They also feel guilty because, as my condition worsens, it becomes more and more likely that I will never be totally independent. I feel guilty because they have to help me in many aspects of my life and it affects their relationship with my sisters. I find myself compensating by not telling them all the things that are bothering me or bad things that have happened. I also feel guilty because they worry about me and because they work so hard just to help me.

As for my sisters, my relationship with them is strained. I think it is strained mostly because they resent me (my older sister more than my younger sister), because they were always sent off to my grandparents' house whenever I had a doctor's appointment, and they viewed it as me getting more attention from my parents than they did. It didn't matter if it was positive or negative attention, because it was still attention. As much as I understand their point of view, I still felt resentful because I felt guilty enough, and have tried my best to not ask for anything from my parents unless I absolutely needed it. But even this seemed to not be good enough for them. As a result, I was always left out and felt isolated. All of these things made me feel even guiltier because my parents always felt they needed to referee, which is not fair, and it has affected their relationship with my sisters a lot.

Even though time has passed and we are older, I still feel isolated and left out. They know all of the things that I have gone through, and I think that they still don't really understand and still resent me on some level. I honestly don't think that the issues we have will ever be resolved, because they are too hurt and I am too hurt. I love my sisters with all my heart and I will always be there for them, but I will never be close to them like I have always wanted. I feel that because of aniridia, I have lost my sisters, and it is very hard to feel like I am going through this without them.

My best advice to new parents of children with aniridia is to explain to your other children early and often what is going on with the child who has aniridia. Get them involved in the process by bringing them to the doctor's appointments. Find a doctor who will answer their questions so that they will understand. And, most importantly, make it abundantly clear to the other children that they are just as important as the child with aniridia. Maybe even try to spend special time with just them (either together or separately). It might help to reduce or eliminate the resentment, and can only add more people to the child's support system.

Beth, United Kingdom—Struggles with Independence

I'm from Manchester, England, and I have sporadic aniridia. I was diagnosed at three months old as my Nana, who looked after me in the daytime while my mum was at work, thought that I was blind as I did not ever open my eyes. I also have nystagmus, strabismus, cataracts, and possibly keratopathy. Currently, I am waiting for a referral to a cornea specialist at the eye hospital. My vision acuity is 3/60 in the right eye and 1/60 in the left eye (in feet it would be 20/400 and 20/800). I used to wear glasses for shortsightedness, but gave up wearing them as they gave me migraines. I also tried contact lenses with painted irises, but my eyes are quite small and it was difficult to find contact lenses that were small enough. I also found the light being focused on a small part of my retina was very uncomfortable and I was more photophobic.

While growing up, I always knew I was different and that I had something called aniridia, but it wasn't until I was sixteen that I found out what it meant or was able to speak to someone with the condition. My parents encouraged me to try the help I was given, and to use it to be as independent as possible. They did not allow my disability to be an excuse for anything. As a result I developed a number of my personality characteristics, including being assertive and determined! I did not have any friends who were visually impaired until I was seventeen. I knew people who were visually impaired, but they were all much younger, so I felt the odd one out sometimes. I did not realize how blind I was until I went to the university. I was in a town I didn't know and with people who didn't know me. I couldn't see to get around, and because I had never been in this situation before I found it difficult to vocalize my difficulties. I ended up with depression and suicidal feelings, and it took me a couple of years to get well again.

This brings me to my biggest struggle. I come from a very small town where I lived in all my life. I was very well known. People knew that I was visually impaired, and I knew the town like the back of my hand. Therefore, my mobility skills in the town were very good. As I said before, at the university I ended up in a city I had never been to with thousands of students I didn't know. I needed to socialize with people, but found that I couldn't see who people were so I would ignore them in the street or couldn't see to find people in the canteen. I had difficulty with my mobility and found it tiring in the daytime, and at night I used to bump into things and fall over. No one helped me find my way around the university until I had fallen down every hole and walked into every lamppost. It took me a while to work out where everything was, including important things like how to get to the local shop. So I asked for some long-cane training for nighttime and at that time I was asked if I wanted a guide dog, but I said no as I thought I could see too much. The guide dogs rehabilitation officer came out to give me some long-cane training. I found it quite useful and tried to use it by introducing my cane as Edna. People name their guide dogs, so why shouldn't my cane have a name? It makes it more approachable. It was still difficult to take on this label of being visually impaired and having people judge me because I was using a cane. I avoided using it when I needed it, at night, as I felt vulnerable.

I also had no equipment as I was waiting for my Disabled Students Allowance to come through so I could get a computer and other support to assist me with my studies. Furthermore, I was in a "Disabled Room," segregated from the majority of other students, which was terrible.

During this time my mental health started to suffer. I was starting to avoid socializing, since it was too difficult to explain my condition to people and why I needed them to guide me or say their name before they spoke to me. I would stay in and eat, and I felt terrible about myself. Then I found it difficult to study. I still managed to drag myself to lectures, even though I spent a lot of time crying and couldn't get out of bed, and as a result I didn't do any of the extra work I needed to do outside of lectures. I had suicidal thoughts and really didn't want to live anymore, since I felt so much pain. I felt that people didn't understand me, and I didn't belong and that I was a freak.

I went to the doctor and told her that I thought I had a problem, and she referred me to an art therapist. I told my mum, who had been concerned as I had stopped taking care of myself and had become withdrawn. She took me home and I commuted to university for the rest of the term. If she hadn't done this, I may well have taken my own life. Luckily I managed to get myself together enough to pass my exams. In the next two years I continued to have therapy and managed to pick up the pieces and move on. My exam results got better and better, and I graduated with a 2:1 in July 2003.

Today I work full time as a community mental health worker for young disabled people. This means that I work with disabled people who have an additional mental health issues, to support them with their mental health on a one-to-one or group basis. Also, I use a guide dog. I have been a guide dog owner for nearly a year now. I have a yellow Labrador called Sandie. I decided to apply when I got my first job, since I found it tiring using a long cane to get around. My social worker asked me if I had applied and I replied, "I have too much sight." She informed me that anyone in the United Kingdom who was blind or partially sighted could apply for a guide dog. I called the next day and put my name down, and went through the application process. The last part of the process was to have a walk with two guide dogs. I walked round the block in an unfamiliar place independently, and I couldn't believe how much easier it was to let the dog make the decisions. I walked much quicker and I was standing up straighter, and didn't have to peer at the ground. Sandie has made such a difference to my life! When it is too sunny I no longer have to squint and peer to see where I am going; I can close my eyes and let her do the work. I know where I am by relying on tactile and audible clues. I don't get migraines when I go shopping, as she negotiates the crowds, and I wouldn't be able to do my journeys to work in the rush hour without her. Getting Sandie was one of the best decisions I have made for my independence, as she has made life so much easier. She is not only my guide but my companion at home too. So my advice to anyone with aniridia or other disabilities is to try to be positive and focus on your abilities. Also, be honest about your limitations, but do not be scared to try things that may seem difficult. Finally, find support in the people who care for you and believe in you.

L.H., United States—Dealing with Bullies

I was born with familial aniridia. My mother and my aunt have it, but not my grandmother. My great-grandfather may have had it, but no one knows for sure. My aunt has two children who did not inherit aniridia, but my brother and I both have aniridia. I also have glaucoma, but it occurred after taking a steroid that I was using to treat a cut gotten from a contact lens. Dr. Netland said I may have had it already, but the steroid caused it to become uncontrolled. My mother, my aunt, and my grandmother have all had cataract surgery. My brother is farsighted and has nystagmus: however, his vision is good enough that he can drive. My vision is about 20/200 without correction. I don't see out of my left eye, except colors (due to the uncontrolled pressure that was caused by the cut), and I see 20/100 out of my right eye with glasses. I am nearsighted, so the glasses are for distance.

I've been through a lot throughout my life, but my most difficult experience was dealing with bullies. They really gave me a hard time. They made my life awful, and I could not wait to get out of school. I was called names, things were thrown at me, and I was pushed, not too hard though, because I would have pushed back. But as a general rule I had an older brother who took care of business if I told him that someone was picking on me. It still happened, but I lived through it. I would not recommend the way I handled the teasing to anyone. It changed me. I rarely talked to anyone. I just wanted to be left alone. I did not participate in anything. You could say I went to school and then I went home. I internalized everything. I still remember the names of the people that harassed me and think about them quite a bit. As someone who went through this hell, all I think about is preventing my children from experiencing the same problem. My main tactic was to ignore the name-calling. I had some people who used to sit behind me in high school and pull out my hair, one strand at a time, or they would throw little pieces of paper in my hair. It was hard to ignore, and sometimes I did say something; however, because of where I live and the kind of people they were, it could easily have led to being cornered somewhere and getting beaten up or worse, so I mostly kept my mouth shut. Now I wish I had slugged them both and taken my chances, but it is too late now. I did graduate and went on with my life, so all is well that ends well, and luckily I had my family to keep me going. I am grateful to them for not letting me do something that would have been destructive to my life. Everyone gave me the freedom to be who I wanted to be and to do, mostly, what I wanted to do. The weekdays were awful, but the weekends made up for it.

My grandfather had a farm, and I got to help there as well as drive a three-wheeler when my brother and older cousin didn't have them. During the summer, I worked at my grandfather's fish market near Kentucky Lake, and no one treated me differently. I got the same amount of work as everyone else. When the factory shut down in the summer, my father would take us to water parks, swimming pools, and to Land Between the Lakes for a day of walking through the coldwater springs and a picnic. I wasn't treated as different when I was with my family, and they helped me to see that being different is not so bad.

As a child I was always losing my glasses, and my dad would tell me that if I would put them in the same place I would find them all the time. I didn't want to find them, and he knew and understood that. He had a hard time with me when I was younger, because he could not comprehend what I could and could not see, but he was a great father. So I believe a strong, supportive family is the key to fighting bullies and teasing. If society would stop being so close-minded, maybe I (and others too) wouldn't be so self-conscious about my eyesight. When I tell a person about my condition, I really don't like the barrage of questions I usually get. I have found that telling people that I can't see very well is a necessity, though: for example, if they wave at me and I don't wave back, or if they ask me to do something and I can't (like drive to their house). I have also found that they look and talk to me differently than before they knew about my disability. I want to be considered just like everyone else, and telling people about my eyesight seems to do the opposite. People need to learn to treat others with disabilities as they do people in their own family, because we're not different and shouldn't be treated differently. We should be accepted and treated the same as anyone who does not have a disability.

C.H. & S.H., United States—Employment Struggles; No limits for Child

I'm from North Carolina and married to my lovely wife. We have a beautiful daughter who has familial aniridia. I have sporadic aniridia, nystagmus, post cataracts, and glaucoma.

While growing up, I encountered many ups and downs. My parents treated me like a normal child, which helped me become more independent. I was always mainstreamed in the public school system. Overall I did well in school; however, math was probably the most difficult subject because I could not see the board when the teacher was explaining the work. Therefore, I depended on friends to help tell me something, tutoring after school, or once in a while an assistant to help explain the work. In college I played most intramural sports and raced in snow skiing with United Association of Blind Athletes.

I met my wife in college, and we knew there was a 50 percent chance our children would inherit aniridia. So when our daughter was born, we felt a variety of emotions. We just prayed that she could see okay. So far she is doing well, and we know she may have visual limitations; however, she can still lead a normal life. So our advice to other parents is do not limit your child. Let him/her do as many things as possible that everyone else can do.

The most difficult experience in my life has been dealing with employment issues. I graduated with a degree in physical education (K–12) with a minor in music (voice). Immediately following graduating from college, I decided to stay in Raleigh, North Carolina, by myself and try to get a job as a teacher at the School for the Blind. I decided to substitute-teach to gain more experience, which would help me land a teaching job. After substituting for six months and applying for over eight different teaching positions and seven house-parent positions at the North Carolina School for the Blind, I decided that the administration had no interest in hiring me for anything other than substitute teaching. Each time I was turned down for one of the positions, I made sure I asked why I was passed over for someone else. The only answer I ever received was that the other candidates had more experience.

After being rejected from the one place that I thought would accept me first, I decided not to give up and to go try to work in the county school system in Raleigh. I worked in the county school system for a while, and then decided to look elsewhere for other opportunities. I was then hired for a teaching position as a third- through fifth-grade self-contained learning disabilities teacher. When I interviewed for the position, I was told that there would be six boys in the class. After hearing this, I knew that it would be a challenge, because my vision was about 20/400 in my good eye due to my cataract, and that I needed to take classes to become certified to teach exceptional children. Even though I knew that the job would be a big challenge, I was ready to accept it in order to gain the experience I needed to land a teaching job in Adaptive Physical Education. Well, this was the beginning of a huge learning experience.

My first day on the job was also the first day of school for the students. What a way to start a new job. My teacher's assistant had already worked several days and had arranged the classroom as she wanted it. Needless to say, by this time she had the impression that she was the teacher. She had already put bulletin boards up and tried to plan a few lessons for the students. This was her first year working as a teacher's assistant, which made it even more difficult because she had no experience working with students with disabilities. I knew that I was headed for one heck of a year. Just when I thought things were bad, they got worse. After the first few days of assessing the students' needs in each subject, I discovered that each student was on a different level, which ranged from first-grade abilities to fifth-grade abilities. This is when I began making three sets of lesson plans for each subject. By January, the principal had allowed six more boys to be placed in this class, and I was going crazy. My vision was so poor that I was using a visual tech machine to grade and read. The students were having major behavioral problems due to the number of students and ability levels in the classroom. I was so stressed by then that I would dream at night and wake up telling my wife to sit down and be quiet.

By February I knew that I did not ever want to teach a self-contained learning disabilities class again; therefore, I decided not to take the classes to become certified. In February the principal of the school kept popping in, observing my class, trying to figure out why there were so many behavioral problems. Of course, she made it look like everything was my fault, and that the students were misbehaving because of my teaching instead of realizing that there were too many kids in the class and that I was in way over my head with my visual potential. After considering resigning, I decided to struggle through the rest of the year, because I was not a quitter. In May the principal called me in and told me that I either needed to resign at the end of the school year or the county would revoke my teaching license. So of course I decided to resign at the end of the year.

I then decided to look other places for employment and got a job as a shipping and receiving clerk; however, after working in this job for a while, I decided I did not want to work in a warehouse earning minimum wage for the rest of my life. So I started my job search again. This time I was hired as a Christian education/youth director at a Presbyterian church. I was very content with my job until a few problems arose, and one was the church's struggling finances. To make a long story short, I was notified that I was immediately terminated from my job, but would be given a three months' severance package. I was completely shocked, because I had never imagined that a church would ever think about treating an individual this way.

During the three months of my severance package, I looked for various jobs that I was qualified for, as well as retail jobs. I would have thought that finding a job would be much easier since I had a lot of experience, but so far it doesn't seem to be true. I have only had a couple interviews, and none of those have led to anything. At this time I am also going through services for the blind and looking into the possibility of going into the Business Enterprise Program, which is a federal program started by the Randolph Shepherd Act. I am also exploring the possibility of starting a small home business with the help of N. C. Services for the Blind. No matter what happens with my career future, I will always have faith in God that he will be there with me through the good times and the bad. I'd also like to say my parents and my wife have helped encourage and inspire me, because they have always been there to support me whether I was struggling with school, employment, or health issues. Without them, I cannot imagine where I would be or what I would be able to do or would have done.

Renee, United States—Testing in School and Driving

I'm from Tennessee and was born with familial aniridia. My mom has sporadic aniridia and my brother has familial aniridia, too. I also have nystagmus, cataracts, and glaucoma. I was never tested for glaucoma until I was twenty-two years old, and I had pressures in the high twenties. My cataracts grew worse in my early thirties. I had cataract surgery on both eyes, one eye in 2003 and then the other eye in 2004. I personally had no problems after either cataract surgery. My vision was a lot clearer, and I can now see a lot more detail. In my teens I wore glasses. All the glasses did was clear up what I could see. I switched to wearing contacts in my twenties. I liked them better than glasses because they seemed to help me see just a little better than the glasses; however, since I have had cataract surgery I do not wear the contacts. The lenses that were put in my eyes have the same result the contacts did.

Since I was not really aware of what exactly was wrong with my eyes, I basically grew up as a normal child who just didn't see very well. I did everything any other kid did, if it was possible. I also didn't have any of the stress that some kids may have these days with having to go to the eye doctor a lot for pressure checks or using eyedrops. I also never had any surgeries. None of that was present, as we were unaware of the threats of glaucoma or cataracts.

School was hard at times. I went to school in the '70s and '80s. No one was really educated back then on the needs of a visually impaired student. It was like they knew about it, but didn't really acknowledge it very much. I also believe some teachers didn't even know about my eye problems, or if they did, they really didn't care, or thought it was not all that bad. I think I had two teachers in all my twelve years of school who did try to remember me and try to help me as much as they could. That really helped me a lot. I had to find a way to help myself most of the time. If we took notes off the chalkboard, I would always have to find someone to let me copy his or her notes later on my own time. I had to ask for a lot of help from the other students at times. Most of the time the other kids were happy to help me. I was an average student grade-wise.

One difficult experience I do remember is when we took annual tests that tested your year level in each subject: it took me longer to do the tests, since the tests were timed. I didn't think it was fair to me, since I am a much slower reader due my vision. They let me go to the library with the special education teacher to take the test by myself. She read me the questions, too. But since it was the special education teacher, the other kids would tell me I was too stupid to take the test with everybody else. It didn't bother me, because I knew better. I never had special education classes, since I was on the same level as everyone else. I also had an issue in high school where all one teacher had us do was answer questions on a handout. We had to look up the answers in the book. At the end of the class, he would have us trade papers and grade them. I never had time to finish, and I was failing. I told the teacher my problem and he at first said he couldn't help. I got really mad and told him he would have to, and he said no, it wouldn't be fair to everyone else if he let me take the paper home to finish it. I said, well then I'll have to talk to the principal about it, and the next day that teacher had completely changed his teaching style to a way that I was able to keep up with.

I just think that these days it would really help if the teacher of a child with aniridia would be given a packet of information on aniridia, so they could read it and educate themselves on it, then talk to the parents and the student. The teacher and parents should take some time to explain the condition to the entire class. Answer any questions they have, and then they will know that the student is not stupid or anything, that they have an eye condition that doesn't allow them to see as well as others.

The most difficult experience for me to go through was driving. It was really hard when everyone started driving and taking driver's education. I sat on the school bus and cried when I looked out into the parking lot. I knew all my friends were getting in their cars and going home, and I had to ride the bus. Of course, I couldn't blame or hold anything against them because it wasn't their fault, and they had no way to know how it felt for me. It was hard thing to deal with, and I don't know how to make it any easier. I missed out on doing a lot of things, but I had it worse because my mother also has aniridia and she cannot drive either. I basically depended on friends to let me ride with them. I lived in a small town. To be able to work, I needed transportation, but there is no public transportation. I have always had to depend on others for transportation, and it has been extremely hard at times. People who have always had the privilege of driving take it for granted and never stop to think about what it would do to their lives if tomorrow they could no longer drive. When I was twenty-five years old I decided I wanted to get a driver's license with monocular glasses* restriction. I had no support from anyone who knew me. I did, however, manage to get a driver's license. I drove for a while around my little small town. I knew the roads and everything really well, but it was still extremely stressful at all times. I could never drive anywhere else outside of my town. I no longer drive, since it's too stressful for me. I'd like to drive, but I am just too scared and afraid I will cause a wreck and someone might die. So I choose not to drive. Now I mostly depend on family and friends. It is still hard to have to depend on others all the time. Just recently we moved into the city, and I have looked into public transportation.

I have found that dating or just meeting new people is hard for me. I hide my eye condition until people get to know me well enough to understand that my eye condition doesn't define who I am. Most people who do not know you, when they meet you for the first time and hear that you are legally blind, they are going to prejudge you somewhat. This is not fair, so I've always felt that I had no choice other than letting someone get to know me first, then telling them, so they can see that it wasn't as big a deal as they may have thought.

Finally, I just want to say that, since I was never treated as if I could not do all the same things as all the other kids while growing up, I grew up a very independent person. I am afraid that if parents of children with aniridia do not understand this, and they shelter them or are afraid to let them try things on their own, that they will grow up not knowing how to be independent, but will be dependant on everyone else for everything.

Brittany—Making it through Public School and Surgeries

"Your daughter will never make it through public school," the professionals told my parents twenty-three years ago when I was born. When I was born, I was diagnosed with aniridia. I was considered legally blind and had three cataracts in my left eye and two cataracts in my right eye.

---

* Editor's note: Please understand that any mention of the use of bioptic monocular glasses for driving does NOT mean that all people with aniridia are candidates to use these devices to drive. Nor do all states allow bioptic glasses for driving.

As I was growing up, my parents were determined that I would go to public school and live a "normal life" along with a visual impairment. To fulfill a "normal life" as a child, I attended dancing, swimming, soccer, and any other type of socialization that a non-disabled child would be involved in.

In kindergarten, I was enrolled in a small-town school in Wyoming. At that time, there was no proper special education program in place. Furthermore, my kindergarten teacher would place me into a rice box (similar to a sandbox) to let me play alone as she taught the other "normal" students. To this day, I believe that teacher was intimidated, unaware, and uneducated on how to teach a child with special needs.

My elementary school years were difficult and frustrating. I worked intensely with the special education teacher and the speech therapist, since they told me that I had a learning disability in English and writing along with my visual impairment. These educational labels did not stop me from doing well in school, socializing with friends, and being an active child. I did not realize that I was "different" until fourth grade, when a male classmate called me "Blindy" a few times a week. As older classmates continued to make fun of me, my sister always stuck up for me. One afternoon, my sister and I were walking home as two sixth-grade boys were making some rude comments about my eyes. My sister threw her violin down and walked over to these boys. All of a sudden, one boy hit the ground as she knocked him in the crotch. After that we walked home and never told our parents about that situation. Four years later, my mom found out from the school principal. The school principal never punished either of us because the boy deserved it. After surviving elementary school and working hard to learn my basic skills, I attended junior high school. The junior high that I attended was known as the "tough" school, and still is to this day; however, going to this school was one of the best experiences in my life.

In high school, it was a challenge to keep up with the popular people due to peer pressure. Along with dealing with the social dynamics of high school, I coped with being placed into the lower track for most of my high school years due to my learning disabilities and visual impairment. I hated these years because I felt that the teachers were more concerned about babysitting the students, not teaching the basic skills that I needed to be able to survive in the real world after high school (college or the work force).

I graduated from public school in 2000 and received high honors, with a GPA of 3.86, and was accepted to Montana State University-Billings in the fall of 2000. Within my first year at MSU-B, I realized that I did not receive many of the transitional strategies in high school that would have made college a lot smoother for me. Although I had received assistive technology as I entered college, I lacked the skills to use it. So my last three years of college, I had to retrain myself to be auditory, then visual, typing my papers with enlarged/speech computer programs. Without my assistive technology, I know that I would not be able to professionally function in the real world.

I graduated from Montana State University-Billings with a GPA of 3.82 in the summer of 2004 with a bachelor of science degree in human services with a focus in community resources for disabilities. (I also received *magna cum laude* honors.) I chose this major because I want to help and advocate for people who have a visual impairment and/or disabilities, and to teach them how to advocate for themselves or with the help of a guardian.

After receiving my human services degree, I received two master's degrees in blind rehabilitation studies from Western Michigan University. I graduated in June of 2007 with an M.A. in orientation and mobility specialist (white-cane skills and travel for the blind) and an M.A. in vision rehabilitation therapy (teaching daily living skills and communication for individuals with visual impairments). Then I continued an internship in low vision therapy.

Now I am employed by the V.A. Medical Center as a low vision therapist. I am thankful for all of the experiences that I had to go through to get where I am now. Life never seemed to be fair as a child, but it has been worth every minute. I have been given the gift of sight because of my generous tissue donors. I will never meet their families, but I am so thankful for their choice to say yes to organ and tissue donation. They gave me not only my sight back, but the confidence to help others with visual impairments. I use my life experiences along with my educational knowledge to teach low vision skills to patients to help them become independent and feel that they can live their life using their highest abilities.

I want to say thanks to my family and all the people who challenged me in school and life to help me discover my passion and to accept my visual impairment. Life has been a struggle, but I feel like I have learned so much. I want to help as many people as I can to let them know that life does continue to the fullest, you just see the world in different ways. It is not so dark any more; it is full of colors and opportunities!

In conclusion, some professionals might tell you, the parent, that your daughter or son will never make it through public school; however, never say never. The most important thing to keep in mind is to have a voice for your special child and teach them how to use their voice. It is amazing to me to see the other side of ignorance as an educated college student. There are professionals out there just like my kindergarten teacher who do not have a clue. They might be book-smart, but without the experience, they will never empathetically understand a child with special needs. Determination is empowerment, ignorance is bliss, and self-advocacy is a tool for a lifetime.

Terry, United States—Communication and Understanding

I was born with familial aniridia, and I also have astigmatism, nystagmus, cataract, and recently "floaters." Only in the past several years have I realized that everybody has some issues they must deal with. There is no shame in having a problem, only in not doing what you can to accept or fix it. Being more open helps others know about you and how to interact with you. The most important thing I have learned is that understanding and communication is the key. Everybody is different. People need to understand their own conditions, and be ready to tell medical staffs what they experience. Doctors need to realize that their training and experience is valuable, but should be adjusted based upon patient response also. The more open and honest communication is present, the smoother the ride will be for everyone. It is also important for any disabled person to communicate to their family and friends what help they need. Family and friends should respect those wishes and do things as the person requests. Basically, we should treat everybody else in a decent, respectful manner and just try to get along as best we can. This is why the Aniridia Foundation International is so important, because it gives individuals, families, doctors, and professionals the information and support they need. It helps people cope with feeling like an outsider and not knowing where to turn for help. As for me, I became more at ease with my own condition by watching other people with more severe problems to deal with in life. There are many people who don't come to terms with their condition on their own like I did.

Amy, United States—Life Lessons

I was born with aniridia and low vision. My vision is 20/200. Living with a disability has been a challenge. One thing I have come to realize, though, is that everyone has something that disables us from having a "perfect" life. Be it physical, emotional, mental, or spiritual, we all face some type of adversity. The big question is, what do we do with it?

When I look back at my childhood, I view it as "normal." Of course, there were obvious differences between myself and the other kids, but I do not remember anything that was just extremely devastating! My parents might remember things, but I don't. I do remember sitting in the front of the class if not up by the teacher in front of the blackboard. I have noticed throughout the years that if I am comfortable with my vision, then most of the time others are, too. I attended public elementary schools. During those years, I received large-print textbooks from the school system to use. I was also given large-print achievement tests and given more time to do the tests. I played out on the playground just like everyone else. I've always enjoyed being outside and active.

Toward the end of my fifth- and sixth-grade years, I began to have problems with my eyes. They would wear out after reading a lot with a magnifier. By junior high school, I was having trouble getting my eyes open in the morning. They were always tired and just felt better closed. My parents made the decision to home-school me after my seventh-grade year. They decided that it would be best since I was having so many problems with my eyes.

At that time, I hated the idea. I mean, really hated it. I was afraid I wouldn't have any friends to do things with or talk to. Looking back, that was crazy, but at thirteen or fourteen years old, those things are very important! When I think about the bad attitude I had, I cringe. My mom did the teaching. She read everything to me because of my eye problems. Well, to address the worry of having no friends, throughout the five years of home schooling, I did many things with other home-school teenagers, and had social interaction at church. I didn't lack socially at all, and guess what, my friends didn't abandon me! I also had a graduation ceremony just like "normal" teens! By the time of graduation, I was so thankful that my parents had decided to home-school me. I know what you are thinking: wow, big change of attitude! Throughout those years I developed such a bond with my mom, and I was able to do many things that I wouldn't have had the opportunity to do in a traditional setting.

The next step was college. I had the idea of going away to a school that I had visited with a friend for fun. During high school, I really didn't think much, if at all, about going to college. However, a visit to the campus of Blue Mountain College started my mind in motion. I believe we went down for the visit either my sophomore or junior year of high school. At that time, even though I knew I was interested, I didn't dare say anything. I thought, "This is crazy! My parents will never go for this." But even with all those thoughts, I knew God had led me to that school for a reason.

During my last year of high school, we started talking about college. I noticed the college talks were all centered on schools in town. I thought, "What am I going to do?" I started dropping hints about going off to school. I remember talking with my mom one night. I told her what was in my heart. She said, "Well if you feel like that is where God is leading you, we will check it out." She shocked me! Within the next few months we went down for a visit, and then I applied. I was accepted!

I spent four years at Blue Mountain College in Mississippi. I lived on campus, but it was close enough to come home on the weekends if I so desired. I learned many things. It was a very hard step for me to leave my comfort zone. I faced many challenges throughout those four years. One in particular left me seriously wondering if I could successfully make it through. During those tough times, I clung to my faith in Jesus Christ. I knew that God led me to Blue Mountain for a reason. I learned many things and met many good friends. I learned, for example, that I have to get my pride out of the way and just ask for help when I need it. When I first moved there, I'm not really sure what my logic was, but I just went on living like there was nothing different about me. As time went on, I noticed many things that I needed help with. My vision at that time had decreased to 20/400. Throughout the years I learned humility, and the lesson of not being so hard-headed and independent. The crazy part is that there is absolutely nothing wrong with asking for help if you need it. I would be more than happy to help someone, so why wouldn't I ask for help? Well, I can honestly say that by the end of those four years, I was comfortable with asking for help if I needed it. I'm not saying it's always easy, but it is much easier for me now.

After surviving college, the famous question of "What now?" arose. I wasn't exactly sure what type of job I wanted. I was thinking, I just need a part-time job, so that I can make money but still have time to have fun! I enjoy listening to contemporary Christian music, so I thought I should get a job at a Christian bookstore. My logic was that I would find out about new music and get a discount on stuff. Well, great ideas, but where was reality? I mean that could happen, but that's not what God had in store for me. Those were *my* plans.

I visited a bookstore where we knew an employee. She said I would have to look up items on the computer a lot. I looked at their computer screen. There was a problem: I just couldn't see it. I left disappointed, but it was the months to follow that were hard. I thought, "I'll never be able to get a job, so I'll have to live at home forever and it will just be horrible." Living at home is not bad at all, but everyone gets the urge at some point in their life to go out and conquer the world. I also knew that I would go out of my mind if I continued to sit at home all day, every day. So my parents and I started praying that God would lead me to a job that was right for me. There were certain things that we prayed for. I desired to work somewhere close to home, because I can't drive. I was also concerned about getting equipment that would help me visually. I placed all my concerns in God's hands, because I knew that He had a plan. My "job" at that point was to sit back and trust Him.

There is an agency here called Clovernook Center for the Blind. They have a program called Job Development. I had heard of this before, but my thoughts on it were, no way. I had this attitude because my interpretation was that they have a certain job and just stick you in it. Well, I was wrong. The program was explained to me. With a new understanding, I decided it was something for me.

Jeni from Clovernook handled my case. We met a few times. We discussed my background and interests, and then she helped me look for jobs that would fit those things. Within a few weeks, she scheduled a job interview for me. Talk about stress and anxiety! Now, here I am praying for a job, Jeni finds one, and I start to panic? My thoughts were, "This is too quick, what's going on?" Jeni was great though! She was always there to say, "I promise, you will be okay. You can do this." She helped me prep for the interview, drove me there, and helped me fill out paperwork. I was very nervous, but I survived. I received a call that afternoon with the job offer. I said I would think about it and call back tomorrow. I knew I would take the job, but I was overwhelmed that it all happened so fast. There are moments in my life where I am concrete in my faith. I pray about situations and trust God to make things happen. Then when it happens, my flesh takes over. I start thinking, "Are you sure about this, God?" It's always a problem when I start thinking instead of totally trusting. I am thankful that God is patient and always reminds me that He knows best. As I mentioned earlier, I prayed for a job close to where we live. I also prayed for access to equipment that would help me visually. This company was located only five minutes away. They were also willing to provide any special equipment I would need. I accepted the job and have now worked at Community Services Network of West Tennessee, Inc., as their administrative receptionist since January 2001.

Throughout the years, I have learned many difficult lessons. Sadly, some have not been *completely* learned. One area has been contentment. I may not have everything that I want, or have everything my way, but God has made things and situations to be the way they are because in His wisdom it's what I need. For example, the issue of being able to drive was a big struggle for me. Like all other teenagers, I looked forward to getting my license and having more independence. However, because of my vision it would not happen for me. It took six years to get past the anger, grief, and frustration to the point where I was "okay" with not being able to drive.

When I was a teenager, a lady suggested that I pray for God to heal my eyes. I was open to the idea and I fully believed that God could do it. In my heart, I already felt that it wasn't God's plan to heal them, but I thought, why not? I prayed for God to heal my eyes, but my heart was still sure that it wasn't in God's plan. The idea of God healing my eyes got me thinking. My true desire was for God to heal my heart more than my eyes. From that day on, I asked God to make the vision of my heart better so that I could see Him clearly.

One verse that has meant a lot to me over the years is 2 Corinthians 12:9–10—"And He said to me, 'My grace is sufficient for you, for my strength is made perfect in weakness.' Therefore most gladly I will rather boast in my infirmities, that the power of Christ may rest upon me. Therefore I take pleasure in infirmities, in reproaches, in needs, in persecutions, in distresses, for Christ's sake. For when I am weak, then I am strong."

My visual impairment has caused heartbreaks and difficulties, but they have made me into who I am today. As I stated before, each of us has things that make our life difficult. We all have heartbreaks. I have learned many lessons through mine. For example, my hands are too small to hold it together. Just when I think I have fixed a part, another piece falls through my fingers. But when I give my broken heart to God, it fits in the palm of His hand with plenty of room to work. He mends all the pieces back together. In my life, I will inevitably have more adversities and heartbreaks. I pray that I will remember to give them all to God. It is also my prayer that when I look at the mends, they will be reminders of God's presence in my life and not memorials of past pain.

It is my faith that keeps me going from day to day. God gives me peace, hope, and joy. This is the reason I can live each day and know that no matter what comes my way, everything will be okay! I would like to thank my family and friends for all their support and prayers throughout the years. I would also like to thank you for reading my story.

Barbara—Surgeries

Transplant and *surgery* are scary words individually. Put them together and they are even scarier. Yet, to have a chance, a hope, a possibility that this frustrating, frightening, and limiting vision loss can be stopped is so appealing. Maybe I'd even get some of the lost vision back again. It was such an emotional struggle facing the decision whether it was better to have the surgery with all the possible problems or to continue losing my vision with no other hope on the horizon

It's scary to lose your vision. I didn't know how I was going to be able to get by in life with just the basics of taking care of myself, much less how I'd deal with all the other life activities which I've enjoyed and become attached to over the years. I had known for a long time that having aniridia could possibly cause me to lose my vision eventually, but my vision had been fairly good and relatively stable most of my life. Then suddenly I started having a noticeable decrease in vision every six months. Something had changed, and I had to start facing the reality of losing my vision much more quickly than I had ever expected. As each six months went by, I found that I had to limit my driving more and more, until I finally had to give it up. Now I was dependent on limited public transportation and other people to get to and from work and activities.

Living in the suburbs of a big city where friends and activities can be scattered over many miles and significant travel time, I found that I had to give up activities I enjoyed because I could not get there. I could no longer meet a friend for lunch or dinner because I couldn't get there. The only activities I could do were those that my husband and I could do together. I was so grateful to have him and his willingness to accommodate my vision loss, but I also felt guilty that he had to give up his freedom as well. He always had to worry about taking me places and being subject to my work and activity schedule. He gave up activities in which I could not participate as well. My options in our major avocation, community theater, became more limited as I could not get to rehearsals unless we were both cast in a show. Then it became almost impossible for me to get cast anyway, since I could not read a script to audition. I was frustrated and facing major changes in my life. While I knew that I would adjust somehow, and that I'd still be able to get by and find things to enjoy in life, I knew that those things would not include the activities I had come to love over the years.

There was this surgery called "corneal limbal stem cell transplant surgery" that held out some hope of stopping the deterioration and maybe restoring some of the vision; however, the risks of transplant surgery and the risks of making the eyes worse instead of better were very daunting. There are always risks in surgery, and if something goes wrong, the eye may be damaged in some way. Even if nothing goes wrong, I might go through all the pain, cost, and risks and end up back where I started if my body just rejected the transplants. I might go through all of it and end up with other health problems caused by the side-effects of the immune-suppression drugs. I'd had experience with the steroid prednisone, used as one of the immune suppressants, and it hadn't been a good experience. So many possible side effects, and it is so very difficult to predict how any individual is going to react in advance. It's a huge risk to quality of life in non-visual aspects. Plus, there are many costs in time, money, and emotional turmoil. So many doctor visits, trips to Cincinnati for surgery and check-ups, expensive medications, and never knowing from one day to the next what life will be like. Carrying the risk of rejection of the transplant with me through the rest of my life was scary, too. There was no way to tell if it would all be worth it beforehand, and once started, I'd have to carry on through the process.

In the end, after thinking through this decision for a few months, I realized it all came down to one bottom line: Go blind in the next few years or take the risk of surgery. Those were my choices, plain and simple.

This decision must be a highly personal one, because each option has its own issues and neither is ideal. For me, when I gave myself those two basic options, it became very clear. I really did not want to go blind and lose the abilities that I had. I had invested too much of myself in theater, in dancing, in crafts, in becoming more social. I could not give up those things without a fight. Sure, I could have redirected my energies or found ways to participate in a limited fashion, but it just hurt too much to have to watch other people doing the things I wanted to do and couldn't, only because I could not see well enough. It hurt too much to know I had the ability, knowledge, and skill, but not the vision. I would have had to give up those activities completely and find whole new activities, interests, goals, and dreams, because it hurt too much to be exposed to the loss of what I had worked so hard to achieve. I had to take the risk and try. For me, it was the only choice that worked.

After making the decision to proceed with the surgery, I had to wait several months for the scheduled surgery date. Waiting was hard because after the emotional struggle to decide, I was ready to get started. I didn't want to live with the poor vision. Of course, I didn't know then that I would have to pass through months of pain and worse vision before seeing the real results of the transplant.

I spent the waiting months getting my life and myself ready. I wanted everything organized, cleaned, and paid in advance so that I wouldn't have to do much for a month after the surgery.

When surgery finally arrived, I was very nervous. I was about to start down an uncertain path that held both hope and struggle. The voyage to stabilize my vision that would dominate our lives for more than the next two years was about to begin. My family and friends were so very supportive that I had the courage and confidence to go through with this. They made me understand that whatever happened, they would be there for me and we'd deal with whatever happened in the best way possible. That ongoing support was what got me through the long experience with all its roller coaster–like ups and downs.

The recovery time for this surgery is about three months. I hadn't believed that it would take that long. It turned out to take much longer to see the results. The first surgery was difficult for my body physically. With an eye so swollen and painful that I had to sleep sitting up for weeks, and pain that was not controlled by a full dose of pain medication, the first few weeks after surgery were difficult to endure. But despite the pain, the improvement in the vision gave me much hope. With the scarring removed from the surface of the cornea, my vision was clearer and I no longer saw multiple images. I could tell that my vision would be clearer even through the swollen eye after the bandage was removed and the eye gently coaxed open the morning after surgery. I couldn't see very well that day, but there was a noticeable difference. The surgery had gone well and the eye was recovering fine. Everything was encouraging. But after four weeks, I woke up one morning to find the eye very red and the vision worse. Rejection had set in.

Medication levels are different for each individual, and the doctors have to monitor blood levels carefully. Well, it turned out that my body is unusually good at getting rid of one of the immune-suppression medications, Prograf. The amount I was taking, which would be fine for most folks, was way too low for my body. There just wasn't any way to predict this.

Treating rejection involves putting Pred Forte drops in the eye every hour and increasing the oral prednisone dose significantly to suppress the immune reaction as quickly and completely as possible. Over several days, the irritation in the eye from the drops became rather painful and the side effects of the oral medications difficult. Despite that, I followed the doctor's instructions carefully, because I was driven to do whatever I needed to do to make this opportunity to restore my vision work.

We saved most of the transplant by treating the rejection immediately, and had hoped that the new stem cells were still completely healthy. Six months later, though, my vision had returned to about the level it had been at before the surgery, because there was enough weakness in the ring of stem cells to allow my own bad stem cells to put bad cells on the cornea surface again.

So, eleven months after the first transplant, I was in for a second transplant on that same eye to replace the two bad sections. Because I was already on the immune suppression regime, this surgery was much less painful and I recovered much more quickly. I also knew what to expect and had learned some valuable lessons on how to care for the eye and myself after surgery. The transplant on my other eye, nine months after that, was also much easier.

During my recovery from both my first two transplants, I had setbacks where I developed a hole or tear in the cornea surface. Luckily, in both cases, this did not affect the health of the stem cells, and the surface healed after a few weeks. There was more pain from the drops, though, and it did slow down the recovery. I learned that the surface really is delicate for the first couple months. Taping the eye shield to my face whenever I sleep, using snorkeling goggles to shower, and being very gentle when touching the eye is important for several weeks.

Patience is important in this whole process. People ask when I'll know what my vision will be like, and it's hard to explain that the new surface on the cornea takes three months or more to even out and settle down. That even after the surface is well healed, we have to evaluate what else may or may not need to be done. The stem cell transplant is not always the only surgery needed. Recovery takes patience, as I can suddenly experience a pain episode at any time. The dried drops and mucus in the eye collect around the stitches and break free. My energy level and medication side effects can vary considerably from day to day. In the first couple of months after surgery, all my commitments were made with a "if I'm up to it" caveat. It takes patience to wait to see how the eye will heal and stabilize. Doctor appointments are scheduled based on current progress, so advance planning is difficult. The exact course of future treatments depends on the results of the current treatment, so when the process starts, it is not possible to predict exactly what surgeries or treatments are necessary or a realistic schedule for them.

In my case, after my second stem cell transplant in my first eye, I developed a bad cataract from the topical steroids. I hadn't seen dramatic improvement in the vision after the second transplant. It was somewhat depressing, but I suspected that there was a cataract forming. I was right, and it accelerated over the next five months. I needed cataract surgery, which improved my vision in that eye from 20/800 to 20/80.

That was when the results of the surgeries really finally came through. It took a couple months for my eye and my brain to readjust to this new situation. It had taken eighteen months and three surgeries, but I was finally able to feel like I could return to doing activities that I had given up because of my vision. I started to have hope that I'd be able to live without depending on other people and assistive technology for many things. Most wonderfully, I could see people's faces again. Just being able to recognize people and to see them while talking to them made me feel so much more a part of life again. I could read a restaurant menu, the temperature dial on the oven, a newspaper, or a book without a magnifying glass. I could now read the signs in the subway stations, so I'd know where the train was and could get off at the right stop. I could walk around without fearing that I'd fall down the steps or off a curb because I didn't see them. All these wonderful, trivial things that make life easier. My doctors may not know it, but I thank them every day.

When the vision was 20/80, we decided that that was functional enough that we did not want to risk a cornea transplant in my first eye, even though there is some scarring in the lower levels of the cornea. With my vision at a reasonably functional level, the risk of rejection with a cornea transplant, which is more invasive and more prone to rejection, was not worth it.

I've had the stem cell transplant on my second eye and the vision has improved from 20/400 to at least 20/160. There is still some fogginess in the cornea and probably some cataract too. I don't know yet what other surgeries are in my future or where the vision in this eye will stabilize. I don't know if I'll successfully taper off the immune suppression over the next few years without rejection. The transplants could be rejected at any time. That's scary too. But despite the pain and uncertainty, I am happy for each day that I can see this well.

Alison, United States—Finding Employment

My name is Alison and I'm 28 years old. I was born in Pennsylvania Hospital in Philadelphia, Pennsylvania, and I currently live in Lafayette Hill, which is a suburb of Philadelphia. This is where I have lived my whole life. I was born with sporadic aniridia. I also have glaucoma, nystagmus, ptosis, and corneal pannus. Right now I am working for my uncle part-time. He owns a locksmith business, and I have been helping out with the office work. It is not what I went to school for, but I have not been able to find a job in my field as of yet. All my life my parents treated me like any other kid. I was not treated differently just because I could not see as well as the other kids. I played outside with the neighborhood kids riding our bikes and skating. We ran around and chased each other. I was always a very quiet kid. I did not have many friends. I stuck with a small group of people whom I felt comfortable with.

Before I joined Aniridia Foundation International (AFI), I felt alone. I knew I had my family and friends to support me, but they couldn't truly understand all the things I was feeling. When I met the people from AFI and started talking to them, I really felt like they understood what I meant when I said certain things. I also felt good to know that I can answer parents' questions about a child who has just been diagnosed and make them feel a little more hopeful about the future.

I have tried to explain aniridia to others. Some people are very open and listen to what I have to say. Others are very close-minded. For example, when I went to Aniridia Foundation International's medical conference in Memphis, Tennessee, a few years back, I was in the elevator on my way to one of the events. I was wearing my yellow T-shirt that we all bought, and a lady in the elevator with me asked me what the group was for. I told her we had aniridia and that we do not have an iris in our eye. Her response was asking me and my husband who she had to stay away from to not be affected by aniridia. So I am comfortable telling people who really want to listen about what is wrong with me, but when it comes to ignorant people, that is when I say forget it, you are not worth it.

During my life I would say the most difficult experience so far has been getting a job. I have my B.S. in psychology: cognitive rehabilitation, and my M.A. in clinical health psychology. I have had experience during the last year of my bachelor program and in my master's program working in the field. I submit resume after resume, and sometimes I don't even get a call back. Other times I actually get an interview and I think it has gone well, but I will not get a call back from that. The times I have called back to check on the status of the interviewing process, I have been told that the position has been filled. Some have told me it is due to lack of experience in the field, and one man actually told me that I am "grossly overqualified" for the job. So I can't win. I personally think it is because in the field of psychology, eye contact is very important, and that is very hard for me. It is hard for me to keep my eyes open fully, partly because of the light and, even when they are open, because of my drooping lids it is not always clear that my eyes are open. They will never say it is because of this, but I have always had and always will have my suspicions.

Throughout my life, my family has always been my inspiration. They never treated me like I could not do something. Even in first grade when my mom went to the Individual Education Plan (IEP) and was told I may never ride a bike or play outside with the other children, she always knew that I could do whatever I wanted to do. The one story I always will remember is about the day I was born, when my parents were told that I had aniridia, and they were upset. My father left my mother that night in the hospital and went to the car, and the first song he heard on the radio was Stevie Wonder's "Isn't She Lovely." Up until this day we always think of this as my song. It helped to lift his spirits and started him thinking that I would be able to do anything I wanted to do.

Throughout my life, if there was anything I wanted to do, they always let me try it at least once. When I wanted to try horseback riding, they said of course. They did not know if I would be able to do it, but I did and I loved it. I have come so far in life because they believed in me. They never told me no. My sister has also played a big part in me coming so far. She loved school (for some odd reason). Knowing it was not my favorite thing, she would always help me with my homework if I needed it, even though she was younger than me. When she did better than me at things, she never made me feel bad about it. She was always there telling me I would do better next time. We fought like any two sisters do, but in the end we always knew that it was just over something stupid and we would always be there for each other.

Matthew, Canada—Four Generations

The Bowers family has dealt with the condition of aniridia for many decades now. It began with the birth of my grandfather. Before him there had not been an instance of the condition. Many different assumptions were made, and since genetic studies still had a long way to go, any explanation was homegrown and paved by speculation for generations to come.

My grandfather had five children, three males and two females. Three of them were affected by aniridia. The first-born and last-born were not affected by aniridia, but both utilize corrective lenses for everyday use. Of the middle three, two are male and one is female. Each has led his or her own independent, fruitful life.

My grandfather attended the Oklahoma School for the Blind. There he was industrious, involved, and a mentor to younger students. Following that he attended and completed trade school. He survived the "Dust Bowl" and picked fruit in California. All in all he faced the adversities that many visually impaired individuals did in that time. Being labeled didn't stop him from being a great engineer of all things mechanical and a successful business owner. He wasn't about to let his limitation stop him, and he passed that on to his children.

His daughter excelled academically, attending her father's alma mater for high school and then completing university in her home state. She later became a strong voice for visually impaired individuals. In time, local and national organizations were fortunate to have her as an active member and leader in their advocating efforts. Always a beacon of independence and character, she endured, adapted, and overcame obstacles, viewing each as a personal challenge.

The eldest of the two sons with aniridia followed his father's path in life. He was a mechanical engineer. He was an upholsterer and fabricator by trade. He also owned small businesses. He fathered four children, none of whom were affected by aniridia. Later on in life he underwent cataract surgery and used a system of contact lenses and spectacles that enabled him to access his dream of being independently mobile by driving. Unfortunately, he passed away not long after that.

Then there's my father. He, too, had corrective surgery. This has helped him pursue many things. Just like his brother and sister, he attended his father's alma mater, and then attended college locally. My father has owned small businesses; his determination and hard work enabled him to break through social and professional barriers. He is probably the most intelligent teacher I've ever had. As such, he ingrained his positive attributes and attitude into my sister and me.

My sister was the first in our family to be educated solely through inclusive public education. Her time in public education was very successful and has made her independent. Throughout her schooling she stayed quite involved and was a respected member of her class for her leadership. Her horizon looks promising as she pursues her dreams.

That brings us to me. I attended my grandfather and father's alma mater. I also was mainstreamed back in the mid-1980s, as my sister has been. As a youngster I was involved in the scouting movement. It helped me adapt to living in a sighted world. Those experiences have played a principal part in making me the person I am today. I've always been independent and artistic. I've dabbled in all forms of art, from music, sculpture, painting, and writing, to the culinary arts.

I have fathered one child. My son is affected by aniridia. Though still very young, he shows signs of being very independent, and just as smart as his grandfather. He attends public school, where his teachers say he is bright and well adjusted.

Even though aniridia challenges those who have the condition, it would not be fair or polite to not include those *around* those with aniridia. They are "affected" by the condition as well. They must learn to cope and adjust to life with those with aniridia. It is without question their giving, understanding, love, and positive support that enables individuals with aniridia to lead a productive life.

Our family has been coping with aniridia for four generations. Each generation has witnessed advances in science and humanity. So much more is known about aniridia these days even compared to when I was a child in the 1980s. Also, the acceptance and inclusion of limited individuals as a whole has improved immensely. Our community still has some ground to gain, and vigilance cannot be relaxed. Through continued learning and positive action, the lives of those with aniridia get better.

Jeanne, United States—Misunderstood

My first awareness that I could not see as well as other people happened when I was four years old. A lady came to our house and brought some toys for me to play with. She and my mother sat on the couch talking while I sat on the carpeted floor in front of them exploring the new colorful shapes and objects. I had no interest in their conversation, which revolved around what I could see and what it seemed I could not see. No, I didn't bump into furniture or large objects. Yes, I could see colors well. Yes, I held small objects up close to my face to see them. Yes, my eyes were very sensitive to light and I wore sunglasses when I went outside. After the lady left, and took the toys with her, I asked my mom about her. Mom said I'd be starting school next year and this woman would work with the school and with me to help get whatever I needed to do well in school. I then asked if my older sister and two older brothers, who were already in elementary school, had a lady like that to help them. My mom explained to me that the lady worked with children like me who did not see as well as other people, and so might need extra help. I was content with this answer and walked away, hoping the next time the lady came she would bring her toys again.

As I grew a little older, I would begin to wonder what it was like to be able to see like other people. I thought my vision was just fine. But other people were able to see better. What did that mean? Were colors brighter? Could they see things that I couldn't? It wasn't until I was in first grade that I began to notice the differences in my vision compared to what others could see. Other students could see what was written on the chalkboard, even from the back of the classroom. From the front row where I sat, I saw only a large green rectangle on the wall. There were white marks on the board, but I could not make out any letters or numbers. The teacher would write what was written on the board onto a piece of paper and give it to me so I could do my work. At the end of the school day, students would walk out the door and scan the line of yellow school buses waiting to be loaded. They could see the bus numbers marked on the side of the bus and go directly to their bus. I would need to walk up to each bus in order to see the numbers clearly enough to know if that bus was the one I needed to board. Standing directly in front of the number, about two feet away from the front of the bus, I was close enough to read the black, bold numbers. At first, it took me a while to find which bus was mine. I figured out that my bus was generally parked in the same place every day, so I could walk up to the buses in that area to find my bus. Then one day as I left the school building, I saw someone who rode the same bus as I did. I followed the person and was led straight to the bus I was supposed to get on. I decided this was the best strategy for finding my bus, and from that day on I looked for a familiar person who lived in my neighborhood to follow to the bus.

I discovered on my own the best techniques and methods to use to get around and adapt to the world around me. The lady with the toys worked for the New Jersey Commission for the Blind and was my counselor from the time I was four years old until I graduated from high school. She would visit me at school or at home about twice a year. She provided me with magnifiers, notebook paper with bold dark lines printed on it, and other gadgets that would help me in school. She was a wonderful counselor and advocate. She told me about a summer camp for children who are blind or visually impaired. I spent two weeks every summer at Camp Marcella, the New Jersey State Camp for Blind Children. I went from the time I was six until I was sixteen and could no longer attend. I loved camp. I have many happy memories, met great friends, and learned to swim at camp. It built my self-esteem and gave me the confidence I needed to overcome the challenges and obstacles that sometimes got in the way.

A glaucoma operation at the age of nine resulted in an eye infection and put me in a hospital in Philadelphia over Christmas. Although I lived in New Jersey, my ophthalmologist was in Philadelphia. The eye doctor my parents first took me to when I was six weeks old didn't know what was wrong with my eyes or what could be done. He sent us to a well-known ophthalmologist he had studied under. This doctor diagnosed me with aniridia. He was my ophthalmologist from that first visit until he retired eighteen years later.

So there were and will always be struggles. But because 20/200 vision is all I've ever known, and because I learned to adapt and adjust in a sighted world from such an early age, I've never had the desire to be anything different than what I am. Curiosity is more of what I experienced. What color would my irises be if I had them? What would it be like to hold a book in my lap and be able to read the words, instead of having to lift it up an inch in front of my face before the words become clear enough to read? It is not that I *miss* seeing this way. I have never known vision like that. I can only imagine what it would be like.

I don't like to depend on others for my transportation needs, so I get frustrated mostly from not being able to drive. I don't like depending on a paratransit system to get me to work and back home. A system that provides rides to hundreds of disabled people each day will make mistakes. They will pick me up late. They will drive me around town for over an hour or more while they pick up and drop off other people. Drivers will call in sick or will be running late. A traffic accident from earlier in the day will cause delays. Oh, I do wish I could drive.

Perhaps the most difficult part of living with aniridia for me is being misunderstood. When a person is totally blind, it is obvious that they cannot see. They usually walk around with a guide dog or carry a white cane. A person with partial vision is not usually seen with a cane or guide dog even though their limited vision may allow them to see only a couple of feet in front of them. Certain actions or a nonresponse from someone with a visual impairment can be easily misinterpreted.

When a person waves or smiles at me from ten feet away and gets no reply, I am seen as rude or stuck up. It can appear at times that my vision is much better than it actually is, especially if I am in a familiar environment.

One time I was volunteering at my church fair. The rides set up in the parking lot required tickets. I was stationed at the booth that sold those tickets. I would take money, give change, and give people the number of tickets they purchased. A man came up to the booth with three children to buy some tickets. As he handed me his money, I took the bill and brought it up to about one inch in front of my face so I could see the denomination of the bill in order to give him the correct amount of change. He looked at me and angrily said, "Do you even know what you're looking for?" He was offended because the bill I was looking at represented a large amount of money and he thought I was inspecting it to find out if it was counterfeit. I'm sure from his perspective that's what it looked like. He had no idea I had a visual impairment. Some people will make a comment like that and then just walk away and not give me a chance to explain.

At other times, I try to explain that I can't see well, and then people usually look at me strangely and ask why I don't wear glasses. When I simply tell them that glasses don't help, wanting to avoid a lengthy explanation, people don't believe me. "There must be glasses that would help you, with today's medical technology and advancements. You need to look into it more," they would say. Or, "Have you looked online? The internet has everything these days. I'm sure you could find some glasses that would help you to see better." Total blindness is more common. A person with low vision needing to look closely at an item in order to focus on it and to see it more clearly is rare. People for the most part have never heard of aniridia and are unaware of the unique circumstances surrounding the condition. This can be one of the hardest parts of living with aniridia.

Like others with aniridia, I experience some of its associated conditions. I take eyedrops in my left eye for glaucoma. When corneal scarring began to be present, in his great wisdom, my doctor knew I needed to see a corneal specialist and referred me to one. The progression of the corneal scarring is slow. It is now being monitored by another doctor. He is an excellent, well-known ophthalmologist in the city of Jacksonville. It is comforting to know I am under the care of someone with such expertise in the area of corneal disease. The vision loss I am experiencing is minimal so far. It is good to know there are procedures available now that can restore lost vision from corneal scarring. Much of the knowledge I have about aniridia and the support I receive comes from Aniridia Foundation International, a wonderful organization dedicated to helping individuals and families affected by aniridia.

Presently, I teach special education. I am married. I am active in my church and participate in other groups and organizations. I live a happy and full life. To me, living with aniridia is just part of life, with its struggles and hardships. But I would not be the same person I am today if I didn't have aniridia. I wouldn't know some of the wonderful people I now know. I see the compassion in people, the good-heartedness of people. The outreach and support I have received in times of my eye surgeries is amazing to me. People will stop in the business of their day to show they care. The incredible kindness of people would not be visible and would not have touched me in such a personal way had I not been born with aniridia. Aniridia means the absence of irises, but it does not mean the absence of love, laughter, friendship, and living life to the fullest. My philosophy of living with aniridia has not changed much from the time I was four years old. I continue to accept life the way it is. The hope I once carried, that the lady with the toys would come back, has turned into the hope that researchers and doctors will one day discover new medical advancements to help future generations of people living with aniridia.

Jessica, United States—Acceptance

Before I get started with who I am and the message I want to give you, I need to tell you a quick story. When I was sixteen years old, I met a family that would change my life and my view of myself, and start me down the path to doing this book. I was at my ophthalmologist's office for my six-month check-up. After he examined my eyes and checked my pressure, he sat back and told my mom and I that he had a new patient who was just diagnosed with aniridia at three months old. He went on to ask if the parents of this child could call us to talk, since they were very confused and hurting from the news. My mom and I said, of course they are welcome to call us. That day the father called and came over to see us. He did not bring his wife or their three-month-old daughter, because he did not know what to expect and did not want to upset his wife any more. He sat and talked with us for a while. He was astonished at what I could do and see. My mom put in a videotape of me marching in my high school band. He sat and stared at the TV, saying, "That's you!" I said, "Yes, I've been playing the flute since I was ten years old." He couldn't believe it. He asked if he could bring his wife and daughter back that night. We again said, "Of course." That night when my dad was home from work, the father came back with his wife and daughter. As soon as she saw me, the mother began to cry. I felt awful that she was going through so much, but had no idea what to say to her to make her feel better. My mom sat down beside her and comforted her, telling her several stories of how she and my dad had dealt with my diagnosis. The mother calmed down eventually and listened intently to my mom telling her how she came to realize that I was given to her and my dad for a reason. She asked me several questions and watched the same videotape of me in the marching band.

Before they left, my dad told them something that I'll never forget. He said they never would've gotten through things if I was not such a strong person, because I am one of the strongest people he knows. I stood there trying not to cry and thinking that's not true. I'm not strong, they are the ones that give me strength by supporting and believing in me. As the family left that night, I could see they had realized they and their daughter had hope. It felt good to know that we had helped this family. That just by meeting them, I had given them hope. It was that night that I knew something had to be done to help families like this, since there was not much information on aniridia. Since I have always loved to read and write (I've wanted to be an author since I was twelve years old), I decided I wanted to write a book to help families affected by aniridia. I know what you're thinking: why did it take me so long to get the book going?

Well, honestly, life is what happened. I got so busy with school, and finding a job after college, that I put the book idea on the back burner and kept thinking I'd work on it soon. Then I joined Aniridia Foundation International, and it all finally came together with the help of Jill Nerby and all the doctors. I want to thank the family I met that day for inspiring me to do this book to help others affected by aniridia.

Now, on to who I am. My name is Jessica and I was born with sporadic aniridia and horizontal nystagmus. I'm live Michigan and am married to my loving and supportive husband, Reid. On February 17, 2007, our son Lucas was born with familial aniridia and horizontal nystagmus. My hope for my son is not only that he will be healthy, happy, and to have the most vision he can, but also that he will know he is not alone and there is hope. By being a part of Aniridia Foundation International and reading this book, he will gain experience, friendships, and knowledge that I never had growing up.

All during my childhood I knew I was different, but felt "normal" and just wanted to be accepted as being "normal." I knew I had something called aniridia, but I couldn't explain it to others as I can now. I dealt with bullies all through school. I can remember coming home and sitting on my mom's lap and crying because of all the harassment. I don't remember exactly what they said, I just remember the pain I went through during my childhood. A lot of the time I would take what people said to heart. I would bury it down inside me and let it eat away at me until I couldn't take it any more. I would not recommend this way of dealing with anything to anyone. I learned the hard way that it is not the way to deal with anything.

Looking back at it now, I can see why some of the kids terrorized me. Some had self-esteem problems of their own. Others had bad home lives and just needed someone to take it out on. Everyone is bullied sometime in life about something, but I wish I had known this as a child. It might have helped me accept it more easily. Over time, I've been able to let go of all the hurt they caused me, and I have now left it in the past. I was able to do this because while in college I found and accepted my Lord and Savior, Jesus Christ. Ever since then I have been able to let go of the past and move forward with His comforting arms around me.

I've learned many things during my life, but one that I have struggled with the most is acceptance. Not only accepting myself as I am, but others accepting me for the way I am. So one thing I would like to say to anyone with a visual or any other impairment comes from two things that have helped me through difficult times. One is my favorite song that helped me through some of my darkest days: "Stay the Same" by Joey McIntyre. To me the song basically says "accept yourself for the way you are because it is the way God made you." He made you the way you are for a reason. You may not know the reason, but you need to have faith He is always by your side and will help you through it all. Also, if you have a dream, all you have to do is believe in yourself and you can do whatever you want to do. Look at me, a dream of mine has been to be a published writer, and now I am. If I can accomplish my dream, then so can you.

It has taken me a *long* time, but I finally do believe in and accept myself for the way I am. I feel that aniridia does not define me. It is only one part of me, just like my sense of humor, quietness, stubbornness, and lack of height are a part of me and who I am. Which is why I do not always tell people I have aniridia right away. It is not because I am ashamed at all, but I want them to get to know me a little first before I tell them. Some people react better than others. Some are very understanding and accept me right away. They don't pity me or look at me like I'm strange. But sometimes I don't tell someone because I know I will get a look of pity, a look of "wow, that's weird," or a look of confusion. This is why we need to educate society about eye conditions such as aniridia. It is also why society needs to know and to learn to treat people with disabilities with respect, not ignorance and pity. I know all I want is acceptance from others for who I am and the way I am, not pity or ignorance.

A second thing that has helped me is the word of God. There are several passages that have touched and helped me. Recently, while going through a very difficult trial in my life, I came across a passage that reaffirmed my belief that God made me the way I am for a reason. The passage is Psalm 139:13–14: "You created my inmost being; you knit me together in my mother's womb. I praise you because I am fearfully and wonderfully made." A second passage that has helped me is 2 Corinthians 12:9–10: "He said to me, 'My grace is sufficient for you, for my power is made perfect in weakness.' Therefore I will boast all the more gladly about my weaknesses, so that Christ's power may rest on me. That is why, for Christ's sake, I will delight in weaknesses, in insults, in hardships, in persecutions, in difficulties. For when I am weak, then I am strong." The first time I read this passage, it touched me deep in my soul, and it continues to help me through difficult times. It's helped me realize that even though I am not "normal" in the eyes of society, I am perfect the way God made me. I am glad He made me unique, because without being "different" and going through the trials I have, I would not be the woman I am today. I do not know why He made me unique, but He has a special plan for everyone, and I have finally accepted mine.

5

Glaucoma Problems Associated with Aniridia

PETER A. NETLAND

Glaucoma is a potentially vision-threatening problem that is commonly encountered in aniridia patients. This condition may develop at birth, or shortly thereafter. More commonly, however, glaucoma is acquired later in childhood or even young adulthood. If unrecognized and untreated, glaucoma can result in blindness. For this reason, it is important to be vigilant in watching for this condition in children affected with aniridia. Vision lost due to glaucomatous damage cannot be regained at a later time.

In addition to glaucoma, children with aniridia may demonstrate other problems with their vision.[1] They may have refractive errors, corneal or retinal problems, or abnormalities of eye movement. Foveal hypoplasia (lack of development of the retina) may limit vision in some children. In aniridia patients, cataract (opacification or cloudiness of the lens) is seen with approximately the same prevalence as glaucoma. Cataract, however, differs from glaucoma in that the vision loss due to cataract is reversible.

WHAT IS GLAUCOMA?

Glaucoma is suspected in aniridia patients when there is an increased intraocular pressure. Glaucoma can be definitely diagnosed when changes of the optic nerve occur due to this elevated intraocular pressure. At the later stages of the disease, visual field loss occurs.

In the normal eye, the fluid (*aqueous humor*) in the front of the eye (the *anterior chamber*) is produced by the ciliary body, which is located behind the iris (see Figure 5.1). The fluid produced from the ciliary body flows forward into the anterior chamber, where it drains from the anterior chamber angle through tissue called the *trabecular meshwork*. When there is an abnormal situation, the fluid exits the eye poorly or not at all, and the intraocular pressure may be increased.

The fluid may be blocked from exiting the eye by a closed angle, or may flow poorly out of the eye even though the angle is open (see Figure 5.2). The angle

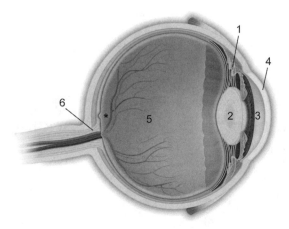

Figure 5.1 Anatomy of the eye pertinent to glaucoma. The aqueous humor flows from the ciliary body (1) around the lens (2) into the anterior chamber (3), which is covered by the cornea (4). Increased intraocular pressure is associated with damage to components of the retina (5) and optic nerve (6). The location of the fovea is indicated with an asterisk. A color version of this figure may be viewed on the companion CD.

(a)   (b)

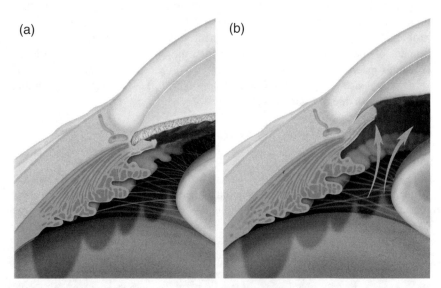

Figure 5.2 In aniridia, the anterior chamber angle may be open (A), but flow of aqueous humor may be impaired in the drainage system, causing increased intraocular pressure. Alternatively, the intraocular pressure may be increased if the anterior chamber angle is closed (B), with the drainage system covered by the remaining iris tissue, which impairs flow of aqueous humor out of the eye (arrows). A color version of this figure may be viewed on the companion CD.

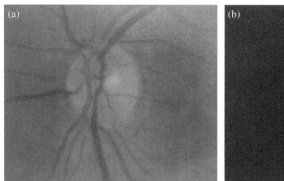
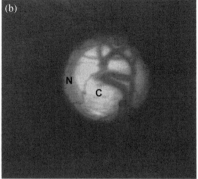

Figure 5.3 (A) Normal appearance of the optic nerve in the left eye of a patient. (B) Glaucomatous damage to the optic nerve in the right eye of a patient. This damage is associated with increased size of the cup (indicated C) and thinning of the neural rim tissue (indicated N). Continued damage of nerve tissue due to glaucoma can lead to loss of vision. A color version of this figure may be viewed on the companion CD.

may be closed in aniridic patients when the stump of residual iris covers the trabecular meshwork in the anterior chamber angle. In some patients, the iris stump does not close the angle, but the fluid still does not flow out of the eye normally. This may be due to a poorly functioning trabecular meshwork, or other problems within the drainage system.

When the intraocular pressure remains at an increased level, damage may occur to the retinal cells, which capture visual images, and also to the optic nerve, which transmits images to the brain. This damage is described as "cupping" of the optic nerve, and means that loss of nerve tissue caused a thinning of the neural rim (the ring of nerve tissue in the optic nerve disc). This "cup" is an empty area that does not contain nerve tissue, because the nerve tissue has been lost due to the glaucomatous pathologic process (see Figure 5.3).

If this damage to the optic nerve continues, visual field loss can occur, usually initially noted in the peripheral visual field. Peripheral visual field defects can be measured in older children and young adults with perimetry, but it is difficult to perform visual field testing on infants and young children. If the process continues, these visual field defects can enlarge and eventually encroach upon the area of central vision, causing loss of visual acuity. This erosion of the visual field, if left untreated, can lead to complete loss of vision. Fortunately, treatments are available that control the intraocular pressure in aniridic patients. With control of the intraocular pressure, the progressive loss of vision can be halted or slowed in nearly all patients. With continued treatment, the chances of retaining vision are good in aniridic patients.

THE PREVALENCE OF GLAUCOMA IN ANIRIDIA

Glaucoma may be discovered either at birth or shortly after birth in aniridic patients, but this is not the most common presentation. If the condition is present at birth, the patients may have enlargement of the cornea (*megalocornea*) or even the entire eye *(buphthalmos)*. There may be small breaks in the cornea, called *Haab's striae*. However, because most patients develop glaucoma later in life, these findings are uncommon in aniridia patients.

The majority of patients with aniridia develop glaucoma in their childhood, adolescent, or early adult years. The reported incidence of glaucoma ranges from 6 percent to 75 percent, but the majority of studies show an incidence of glaucoma of approximately 50 percent to 75 percent in aniridic patients.[1] Therefore, there is a high likelihood of development of glaucoma, but it may take years to develop. For this reason, aniridic patients are monitored for glaucoma from birth through adulthood.

TYPES OF GLAUCOMA IN ANIRIDIA

The glaucoma in aniridia may be due to open- or closed-angle mechanisms. Although there is only a small amount of iris remaining in most aniridia patients, this may fold over the trabecular meshwork, causing closure of the irido-corneal angle by the iris remnant. This angle closure may be progressive, increasing over time.[2] Some patients have elevated intraocular pressure despite an open irido-corneal angle. When the angle is open, there may be no obvious cause for the increased pressure on gonioscopic examination.

EXAMINATION OF THE EYE IN ANIRIDIA

Even if glaucoma is not detected initially, it is important for children with aniridia to have regular examinations of the eye, because the development of glaucoma can occur at any time in childhood. These examinations are directed towards identifying ophthalmic problems that are commonly associated with aniridia.

Even in infants, a complete examination is often possible in the office, without the use of anesthetics. In some instances, a mild sedative, such as chloral hydrate syrup, may be administered. If a complete examination cannot be performed in the office, or when there is uncertainty about the clinical findings, an examination under anesthesia is warranted (see Figure 5.4). Examination under anesthesia does not always require intubation of the patient, as the anesthesiologist may be able to use a laryngeal mask or a face mask for ventilation. Older children (age two to four years) may require an occasional examination under anesthesia to provide good-quality examination of the intraocular pressure and other findings.

During the initial office visit, the examiner will elicit any symptoms, and will question the parents (or the older child him/herself) regarding any visual problems. Often, the classic symptoms of congenital glaucoma, such as *photophobia* (aversion to light), *blepharospasm* (uncontrolled blinking/squeezing of the eyelids), and tearing, are not present in patients with aniridia, who often acquire glaucoma later in childhood. In younger children, it may be difficult to assess the vision accurately, and specialized testing for visual acuity may be performed.

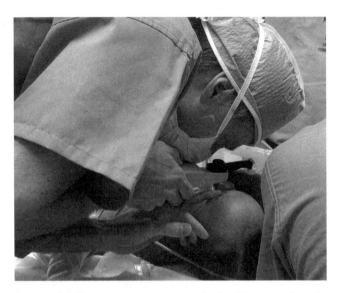

Figure 5.4 Examination under anesthesia. The examiner is checking the intraocular pressure using a Perkins applanation tonometer. A color version of this figure may be viewed on the companion CD.

Usually, a complete ocular examination, including *slit lamp examination* (examination of the front of the eye, with illumination and magnification), *applanation tonometry* (measurement of the intraocular pressure), *gonioscopy* (examination of the anterior chamber angle) using a specialized lens, and *optic nerve evaluations* (with direct or indirect ophthalmoscopy), can be performed in the office in children over the age of five years and, with some training, in children younger than five years. Timing the examination of an infant to occur when the child is placated by a bottle-feeding can allow a complete examination of these younger children.

Visual field examinations can be performed at five to six years of age, but the patient's short attention span and poor fixation often prevent a detailed study. The older and more cooperative the child, the more detailed the examination. By the age of eight to ten years, most children can cooperate for a full visual field examination.

In clinically examining an aniridic patient, the ophthalmologist looks for any abnormalities of the cornea, the clear membrane in the front of the eye that allows light to enter. A slit lamp examination is performed using magnification and a stereo view of the front of the eye. Corneal edema may occur if the intraocular pressure is markedly elevated (see Figure 5.5). In aniridia, over time, a vascular scar membrane—a pannus—may extend onto the cornea. This pannus formation is rare in young children. The lens can also be examined, including an exam for any evidence of cataract (opacification [cloudiness blocking vision] of the lens). Gonioscopy (examination of the anterior chamber angle) should also be performed, ideally using a Koeppe lens, which can look at any portion of the anterior chamber angle. Other types of gonioscopy utilize different lenses with either four or three

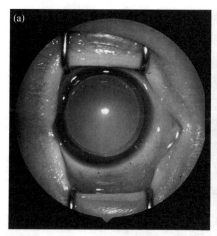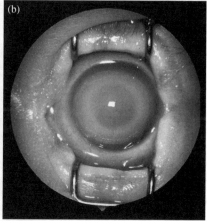

Figure 5.5 Aniridia patient shortly after birth. The right eye (A) has a clear cornea and lens. The left eye has increased intraocular pressure and corneal edema (B). A color version of this figure may be viewed on the companion CD. Reprinted with permission from Mandal AK, Netland PA. The Pediatric Glaucomas. Edinburgh: Elsevier, 2006.

mirrors, which enable the doctor to look at the anterior chamber angle. The patient's vision is measured to determine if a refractive error would be corrected with glasses.

In determining whether the aniridic patient has developed glaucoma, the intraocular pressure (IOP) should be assessed on a regular basis. This measurement of the intraocular pressure (*tonometry*) can be performed with an applanation (usually Goldmann) or by electronic (Tonopen) tonometer. The Perkins handheld applanation tonometer allows the measurement of the intraocular pressure at any angle, including when the patient is lying down. These measurements require a drop of topical anesthetic to dull sensation on the cornea, and then application of the tonometer to the surface of the eye. The intraocular pressure in infants can be measured while feeding or distracted with a pacifier, and older children are usually cooperative if clearly instructed. Children ages two years to three or four years can present the greatest challenge in obtaining accurate IOP readings.

The normal intraocular pressure for a child should be in the mid- to low teens, and certainly not above 20 to 21. Sometimes, because of crying or difficulties in obtaining the measurement, the intraocular pressure may be artifactually high. In this situation, it is important to try to get a measurement of the intraocular pressure under sedation, to make sure that the true reading is not elevated. In children, there is no ideal method of measuring the intraocular pressure. Our preference is the Goldmann or Perkins applanation tonometer, although electronic tonometry (Tonopen), pneumotonometry (a non-contact method, which uses air pressure rather than contact with the cornea), dynamic contour tonometry (DCT), and other techniques may also provide helpful measurements of the intraocular pressure. Applanation tonometry measurements may be influenced by the thickness of the cornea. Studies have demonstrated an increased central corneal thickness in aniridic patients.[3] Increased central corneal thickness could, in theory, influence the measurements of intraocular pressure. Clinicians can try to estimate the effect of this possible artifact.

Another important component of the examination of the aniridic patient is the exam of the optic nerve, looking for any evidence of glaucoma damage. The back of the eye, or *fundus*, is examined using ophthalmoscopy, either in a direct manner, viewing the fundus through with a hand instrument, or with indirect ophthalmoscopy, which uses a light source and a hand-held lens. The appearance of the optic nerve disc is carefully assessed. In the normal situation, the nerve tissue is pink, and there is a small physiologic cup. With glaucomatous damage, the optic nerve may show increased cupping or excavation. If the intraocular pressure is increased, the cup will tend to enlarge irregularly or circumferentially over time, accompanied by thinning of the neural rim.

Cupping of the optic nerve is an early sign of increased intraocular pressure. Evidence of increased cup size is indicative of uncontrolled glaucoma in an individual of any age. Careful drawings are very helpful; also, photographs can be taken of the optic nerve to provide a baseline for future comparisons. Optic nerve cupping occurs much more quickly and at lower pressures in children than in adults. Similarly, in children, a decrease in cupping can occur within hours or days after control of intraocular pressure. This is especially marked in infants below one year of age. In adults, reversal of cupping after normalization of intraocular pressure rarely, if ever, occurs.

Ophthalmoscopy can also be performed to examine the retina. The *macula*, which is the central part of the retina, contains a *fovea*, where there is a concentration of cones and photoreceptors, which give very sharp central vision. This foveal region may be poorly developed (*hypoplastic*) in aniridic patients.

MEDICAL TREATMENT OF GLAUCOMA IN ANIRIDIA

Medical therapy plays an important adjunctive role in the treatment of glaucoma in aniridia. Medical treatment may allow the physician to temporarily reduce the intraocular pressure and improve the clarity of the cornea, which may facilitate surgical intervention by improving the surgeon's view. Occasionally, it may be possible to control the intraocular pressure over the long term with medical therapy. However, in most instances, surgical therapy is usually required for definitive control of the elevated intraocular pressure.

Medical therapies that are commonly used include both topical eyedrops and oral medications.[1] Beta-blocker drops can be effective, but should not be used in children who have asthma or other breathing problems due to possible pulmonary side effects. Carbonic anhydrase inhibitors can be given as drops or as a systemic medication. If the ophthalmologist is concerned that the drop may not be effectively absorbed—for example, because of corneal scarring—the drug may be given as an oral elixir in divided doses during the day. Although safe for pediatric use, oral carbonic anhydrase inhibitors can cause troublesome side effects in some children, such as malaise, fatigue, and loss of appetite. In order to minimize the possibility of systemic side effects, doctors may prefer to prescribe drops, if they can be effectively administered. Prostaglandin analogs are another class of drugs used in reducing elevated intraocular pressure. These drugs can cause mild redness of the eye in some patients, but can be helpful in reducing intraocular pressure.

Certain drugs do not work as well in aniridia. Pilocarpine and other similar cholinergic drugs may not be as helpful. In young children, adrenergic agonists such as brimonidine should be used with caution, as they can cause strong sedative effects. If patients respond well to an appropriately chosen medication, they may be able to achieve good long-term control of the intraocular pressure, and forego, or at least forestall, glaucoma surgery.

SURGICAL TREATMENT OF GLAUCOMA AND ANIRIDIA

Although medical therapy is often tried as the initial therapy, most patients require surgery to provide long-term control of the intraocular pressure. After surgery, however, some patients may still require additional treatment with medical therapy. There are many options for surgical therapy of glaucoma, and the exact choice of procedure will depend upon the specific clinical problems of the individual patient.

Laser Therapy

Laser therapy is helpful in some types of glaucoma, such as adults with angle-closure glaucoma or in adults with open-angle glaucoma. However, in aniridic patients with glaucoma, laser therapies are generally not useful, and are not recommended in most cases.

Prophylactic Goniotomy

Progressive angle closure may occur in aniridia. After monitoring the situation, the ophthalmologist may choose to perform a goniotomy to open the angle and prevent further closure. Thus, further elevation of the intraocular pressure may be avoided. This approach, pioneered by Dr. Morton Grant and Dr. David Walton, can be very effective in preventing the development of glaucoma in some patients.[2,4]

Goniotomy or Trabeculotomy

Goniotomy, described by Otto Barkan in 1936, was reported to be used in aniridia patients in 1953 (see Figure 5.6).[5] The procedure is often helpful in aniridia patients, with the highest success rates reported in young children, usually less than three years old. However, the procedure can be used in older children, particularly those with aniridia, when the angle is observed to be progressively closing. The procedure is performed by making a small incision in the cornea and passing a thin needle-like knife across the anterior chamber to open up the anterior chamber angle and allow the aqueous to flow. Complications due to this procedure are uncommon, especially when performed by an experienced surgeon.

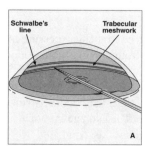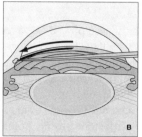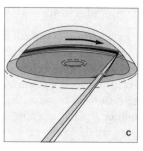

Figure 5.6 Goniotomy. The goniotomy instrument is directed across the anterior chamber (A). An incision is made in the trabecular meshwork in one direction (B) then the opposite direction (C). Reprinted with permission from Mandal AK, Netland PA. The Pediatric Glaucomas. Edinburgh: Elsevier, 2006.

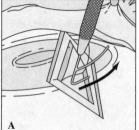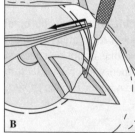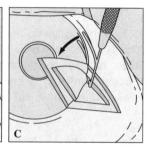

Figure 5.7 Trabeculotomy. After preparation of a partial-thickness scleral flap, the Schlemm's canal is opened with a knife. The trabeculotome is passed into the Schlemm's canal (A), and is rotated (B) in order to pass through the trabecular meshwork into the anterior chamber (C). Reprinted with permission from Mandal AK, Netland PA. The Pediatric Glaucomas. Edinburgh: Elsevier, 2006.

An alternative to goniotomy is trabeculotomy, which is also potentially helpful in patients with glaucoma associated with aniridia (see Figure 5.7). This procedure is useful when corneal edema (swelling and cloudiness) prevents a view of the anterior chamber angle, which is required to perform goniotomy. Some surgeons prefer trabeculotomy to goniotomy because they are more familiar and comfortable with a technique that utilizes the operating microscope. Unlike goniotomy, trabeculotomy does not require passing a knife over the lens, which is not covered by the iris in aniridia. This procedure is performed by making a small incision at the edge of the cornea, and dissecting down to Schlemm's canal. A special instrument, called a *trabeculotome*, is passed into Schlemm's canal, and is used to break open the trabecular meshwork by rotating the instrument into the anterior chamber. This creates an opening that allows aqueous to flow more freely out of the eye.

Goniotomy and trabeculotomy provide very similar results and are very effective. The choice of the specific procedure often depends on the specific clinical situation of the patient and the preferences of the surgeon.

Trabeculectomy

Trabeculectomy is a commonly used procedure to reduce intraocular pressure in older children, or in patients who have failed to benefit from previous goniotomy or trabeculotomy procedures. Initial trabeculectomy may be effective in aniridia.[6] Anti-fibrosis drugs, such as mitomycin-C, are often used to improve the success rate further, because they inhibit scarring, increasing the likelihood of maintaining a patent opening for aqueous flow out of the eye. The average intraocular pressure is lower after trabeculectomy using mitomycin-C as compared with trabeculectomy without this anti-fibrosis drug.

In trabeculectomy, a small opening is made near the edge of the cornea, and covered with small tissue flap. The flap prevents excessive aqueous flow, and thus prevents hypotony (too low intraocular pressure) during the early postoperative period. Later in the postoperative course, once the level of aqueous flow has been determined, the sutures (stitches) used to secure the flap may be released to increase the flow rate through the opening into the drainage area under the conjunctiva (the *bleb*).

In some instances, trabeculectomy may be combined with trabeculotomy.[1] This is a more common procedure in areas such as India and the Middle East, where initial trabeculotomy alone is not as successful. Also, in older children, trabeculotomy may be combined with trabeculectomy if the surgeon feels that a combined technique will give a better chance of success.

Glaucoma Drainage Implants

When other types of glaucoma filtration surgery have failed, or seem likely to fail, the ophthalmologist may choose to use a glaucoma drainage implant. Extensive scarring of the conjunctiva in the area of the *limbus* (where the cornea meets the sclera) following previous surgical procedures is a common indication. In this situation, there is inadequate tissue to support a filtration bleb. If there is a planned procedure around the limbus or the cornea, such as a limbal stem cell transplant, glaucoma drainage implants can be very useful, because they can be performed despite extensive limbal scar tissue.

In glaucoma drainage implant surgery, a small tube is placed into the anterior chamber. The tube drains the aqueous away from the anterior chamber towards the equator of the eye, where a plate is sutured into position. The aqueous drains onto this plate and then flows into the tissues around the plate. The tube, where it exits the anterior chamber and goes back to the implant plate, is covered with a patch graft, often fashioned from donor sclera, pericardial tissue, or some other tissue that resists erosion. The purpose of this patch graft is to cover the tube and prevent it from becoming exposed, avoiding a potential path for infection.

Glaucoma drainage implant surgery can provide long-term control of intraocular pressure in aniridia.[7] As in the choice of other surgical procedures described above, the decision to implant a glaucoma drainage implant is dictated by the clinical history and situation of the individual patient.

Cyclodestructive Procedures

Cyclodestructive (obliteration of the ciliary body, which produces the aqueous fluid) procedures are often used when other types of filtration surgery have failed, or their potential for success is low. The eye may have poor to no vision, or may have the worst vision of the two eyes. If used in a sub-maximal manner (partial or selective ciliary body ablation), cyclodestructive procedures may be used as an earlier treatment option. Extensive cyclodestruction can cause excessive lowering of the intraocular pressure and lead to hypotony, and eventual shrinkage of the globe. In some instances, loss of vision can occur. Sub-maximal treatments reduce the chance of these complications. If other surgical treatments have been performed and the intraocular pressure remains elevated, an adjunctive treatment using a cyclodestructive procedure may be helpful.

THE EXPERIENCE OF SURGERY

Glaucoma associated with aniridia is often treated with surgical procedures. Before any of these procedures, the doctor provides pre-, intra-, and postoperative instructions to the patient's family. Anesthetic drugs enable the patient to remain comfortable during any surgical procedure.

Type of Anesthesia

General anesthesia is used for glaucoma surgery in infants and young children. Great advances have occurred in the safety of anesthesia, and the risks have been minimized. To further reduce any risks, the surgery is best performed at a surgical facility that has familiarity with pediatric surgery.

In young adults, local anesthetics may be used for some eye procedures. In this situation, a sedative is given, and the eye is numbed with local injections of anesthetic. After the eye is anesthetized, the procedure can be performed without pain to the patient.

Recovery After Surgery

Most surgical procedures can be performed as a same-day outpatient procedure, which means that the patient can go home a few hours after the surgery. The patient will be asked to return to the ophthalmologist's office the day after surgery, when the patch will be removed, the vision and the intraocular pressure checked, and postoperative medications started. In most instances after surgery, a topical antibiotic and topical steroid drop is administered to promote healing and prevent infection and inflammation. Usually, these drops are instilled frequently for the first week, and then tapered during the postoperative period.

During the first week or so, the clinician may see the patient several times. After that time, the frequency of checkups is decreased. By four to six weeks after surgery, the eye is nearly healed, and the drops are usually discontinued. When the eye is stabilized, routine follow-up can be resumed.

During the early postoperative period, the surgeon usually asks the parents to cover the eye with a shield, particularly when they cannot supervise the child. This shield protects the eye from any rubbing or damage from direct pressure on the eye. When the eye is fully healed, use of the shield can be discontinued.

There are often restrictions in play during the early postoperative period, intended to minimize any straining, lifting, or roughhousing. Usually these restrictions are reduced two to three weeks after surgery. If the surgeon is concerned about hypotony, the restrictions may be left in place longer. Once the eye is fully recovered, there are no restrictions of activity.

LONG-TERM CARE

In patients who have not been diagnosed with glaucoma, checkups every four to six months during childhood and even into young adulthood are recommended. Frequent checkups are helpful to identify glaucoma at its earliest onset. Early identification can allow timely treatment and prevent visual loss.

In patients who have developed glaucoma and have had treatment for glaucoma, the frequency of follow-up depends on the severity of the problem. If the intraocular pressure is high, or if the patient is recovering from surgery, checkups will be more frequently recommended.

The success of long-term care and treatment is very dependent on the coordination of different ophthalmic specialists. It is important to identify refractive errors and treat any *amblyopia* (lazy eye). Other eye problems, such as cataract and pannus, should be identified and treated as needed. A multidisciplinary approach, incorporating clinical care of the patient, is usually most effective. This multidisciplinary approach includes, not only the ophthalmologist, but also teachers, mobility instructors, low vision specialists, and, of course, the parents.

POSSIBLE FUTURE THERAPIES

The medical and surgical treatments of aniridic glaucoma will, no doubt, continue to improve over time. There may also be new therapies in the future. Currently, stem cell therapy for corneal conditions is possible. Perhaps in the future, stem cell therapy or other treatments for optic nerve problems will be available.

We may also see improvements in the diagnosis of glaucoma in the future. Testing that could identify, in advance, the children who are likely to have problems with glaucoma would be helpful, allowing us to monitor these particular children more closely.

CONCLUSIONS

Aniridia is often associated with glaucoma. Medical treatment may be helpful, but patients often require surgical treatment for aniridic glaucoma. Most of these treatments are effective, so the key to success is identifying the problem early in the course of the disease and preventing damage to the optic nerve. The majority of patients who do lose vision due to glaucoma are not diagnosed in a timely manner, or do not comply with treatment. Therefore, close monitoring is especially important in patients with aniridia. The parents of affected children have an especially important role in seeking out the ophthalmic care that they need to provide skilled and attentive monitoring of their children for glaucoma.

ACKNOWLEDGMENTS

The author is grateful to Mary E. Smith, M.P.H., R.D.M.S., for assistance with editing the text.

Notes

1. Mandal, A. K., & Netland, P. A. (2006). *The Pediatric Glaucomas*. Edinburgh: Elsevier.
2. Grant, W. M., & Walton, D. S. (1974). Progressive changes in the angle in congenital aniridia, with development of glaucoma. *American Journal of Ophthalmology, 78,* 842–847.
3. Brandt, J. D., Casuso, L. A., & Budenz, D. L. (2004). Markedly increased central corneal thickness: An unrecognized finding in congenital aniridia. *American Journal of Ophthalmology, 137,* 348–350.
4. Chen, T. C., & Walton, D. S. (1999). Goniosurgery for prevention of aniridic glaucoma. *Archives of Ophthalmology, 117,* 1144–1148.
5. Barkan, O. (1953). Goniotomy for glaucoma associated with aniridia. *AMA Archives of Ophthalmology, 49,* 1–5.
6. Adachi, M., Dickens, C. J., Hetherington, J. Jr., Hoskins, H. D., Iwach, A. G., Wong, P. C., Nguyen, N., & Ma, A. S. (1997)., Clinical experience of trabeculectomy for the surgical treatment of aniridic glaucoma. *Ophthalmology, 104,* 2121–2125.
7. Arroyave, C. P., Scott, I. U., Gedde, S. J., Parrish, R. K. 2nd, & Feuer, W. J. (2003). Use of glaucoma drainage devices in the management of glaucoma associated with aniridia. *American Journal of Ophthalmology, 135,* 155–159.

6

Cornea and Lens Problems in Aniridia

EDWARD J. HOLLAND AND MAYANK GUPTA

The corneal epithelium is a rapidly regenerating, stratified squamous epithelium. Homeostasis of corneal epithelial cells is an important prerequisite, not only for the integrity of the ocular surface, but also for the visual function. The maintenance of a healthy corneal epithelium under both normal and wound-healing conditions is achieved by a population of stem cells located in the basal layer of limbal epithelium.[1,2] *The Limbus* represents the transition zone between the peripheral cornea and the bulbar conjunctiva. The stem cells from the limbus generate the transient amplifying cells that migrate, proliferate, and differentiate to replace lost or damaged corneal epithelial cells.[3,4] In patients with aniridia, there is a primary dysfunction of these limbal stem cells (see Figure 6.1).

CORNEA PROBLEMS

The cornea is affected clinically in 90 percent of the patients with aniridia.[5] In most cases, the cornea in aniridic patients appears normal and transparent during infancy and childhood.[6,7] However, during the early teens, the cornea begins to show changes. The early changes are marked by the in-growth of opaque epithelium from the limbal region into the peripheral cornea, which represents conjunctival epithelial cells, goblet cells, and blood vessels in the corneal epithelium.[6,7] These changes gradually progress toward the central cornea and may cause corneal epithelial erosions and epithelial abnormalities that eventually culminate in opacification of the corneal stroma, which leads to vision loss.[8] With the gradual loss of limbal stem cells, the entire cornea becomes covered with conjunctival cells. Eventually, many patients develop total limbal stem cell deficiency.

These abnormalities usually become more pronounced with aging. The corneal abnormalities seen in aniridia are collectively termed "aniridic keratopathy".[9] Significant corneal opacification may occasionally be the initial manifestation of aniridia.[6] Abnormal tear film stability and meibomian gland dysfunction are also observed in patients with aniridia.[10] This can lead to dry eyes, aggravating corneal erosion and ulceration observed in aniridic patients.[10] Sometimes,

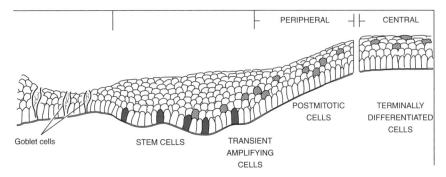

Figure 6.1 A color version of this figure may be viewed on the companion CD. Reprinted with permission of Springer Science and Business Media, from Edward J. Holland and Mark Mannis, *Ocular Surface Disease: Medical and Surgical Management*, 2002.

aniridia is associated with "Peter's anomaly," in which central corneal opacity is present at birth along with defects in the corneal endothelium and Descemet's membrane.[11] The patients with aniridia may have markedly thickened central corneas.[12] This may lead to incorrect estimates of intraocular pressure measured by applanation techniques. Microcornea has also been reported in association with aniridia.[13] Studies in animal models of aniridia have shown that epithelial abnormalities include abnormal corneal wound healing and excessive epithelial fragility. Abnormal corneal wound healing is due to deficiency of matrix metal-loproteinases, while cytokeratin deficiency due to low level of PAX6 expression results in corneal epithelial fragility.[9]

DIAGNOSIS

The diagnosis of aniridic keratopathy is made by the presence of severe epithe-liopathy with corneal neovascularization, absence of palisades of Vogt, and increased flourescein permeability indicative of abnormal epithelial junctions in patients with iris and other ocular abnormalities consistent with aniridia.[7,14] Clinical diagnosis can be confirmed histopathologically by the demonstration of conjunctiva-like tissue on the corneal surface.[7,14]

MANAGEMENT OF CORNEAL PROBLEMS ASSOCIATED WITH ANIRIDIA

In the initial stages when the central cornea still has normal epithelium, treatment is to maximize the health of the ocular surface by treating associated conditions such as dry eyes and blepharitis. Lubricant and bandage contact lens are used for symptom alleviation and for the treatment of recurrent erosions. However, the mainstay of treatment of aniridic keratopathy is surgery. In the past, aniridic keratopathy with significant loss of vision was treated by penetrating keratoplasty (corneal transplantation). Penetrating keratoplasty involves surgical replacement of the central portion of the host cornea with that of a donor eye. The problem with this procedure was the high rate of recurrence because it does not address the stem cell deficiency, which is the primary etiologic factor in aniridic keratopathy.[15] Due to this reason, limbal stem cell transplantation has gained wider acceptance in the management of aniridic keratopathy over the last decade. There are a number of different procedures used for limbal stem cell transplantation based on the carrier tissue (conjunctiva or cornea) and the origin of the donor tissue.[16] The two commonly used techniques are keratolimbal allograft (KLAL) and living related conjunctival limbal allograft. Keratolimbal allograft is the procedure in which cadaveric limbal tissue is transplanted by using the peripheral cornea as carrier tissue.[14] The procedure has two specific advantages over other limbal stem cell techniques. First, stored donor tissue is readily available. Second, keratolimbal allograft affords the largest number of transplanted limbal stem cells compared with any other limbal stem cell transplantation technique[14] (see Figure 6.2a,b). The conjunctival limbal allograft uses conjunctiva as a carrier tissue for limbal transplant.[16] Conjunctival limbal allograft supplies goblets cells in the transplanted conjunctival carrier tissue.[16] However, because aniridic patients have normal conjunctiva, they do not benefit from donor conjunctiva tissue.[14] Moreover, living related conjunctival limbal allograft delivers a maximum of 50 percent of the limbus of one eye, whereas keratolimbal allograft provides up to the equivalent of 150 percent of the limbus.[14] For the above-mentioned reasons, keratolimbal allograft is the preferred choice in the management of aniridic keratopathy.[14]

Human amniotic membrane transplant has also been used for management of ocular surface disease in aniridic keratopathy.[17] It reduces the inflammation and promotes ocular healing temporarily. However, it is not a source of limbal stem cells and therefore not a good long-term solution.

It is recommended that keratolimbal allograft be performed earlier in the disease process. Since aniridic keratopathy involves only the superficial epithelium in early stages, keratolimbal allograft alone may be sufficient for visual rehabilitation.[14] However, in later stages, epithelial keratopathy will typically lead to stromal scarring and the patient will probably need penetrating keratoplasty in addition to keratolimbal allograft.[14] If needed, it is recommended that penetrating keratoplasty be performed after a period of three months from keratolimbal allograft.[14,18] This gives time for the ocular surface to stabilize.[14,18]

Holland et al. conducted a study to evaluate the role of keratolimbal allograft technique in the management of patients with aniridic keratopathy.[14] The study was conducted in 31 eyes of 23 patients with aniridic keratopathy treated with keratolimbal allograft. The mean follow-up time was 36 months, with a minimum postoperative follow-up of 12 months. They found that 23 eyes (74 percent) had a stable ocular surface following keratolimbal allografting.[14] Mean visual acuity improved from 20/1000 to 20/165. Nineteen (90.5 percent) of 21 eyes receiving systemic immunosuppression obtained a stable ocular surface, whereas only 4 (40 percent) of 10 eyes not receiving systemic immunosuppression achieved ocular surface stability ($P < 0.01$). In the 23 eyes with successful reconstruction of the ocular surface, 7 (30.4

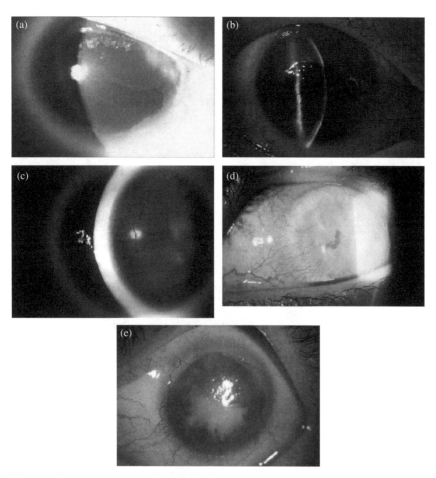

Figure 6.2 (a–e) A color version of this figure may be viewed on the companion CD. Photos represented with permission from personal library of Edward J. Holland, M.D.

percent) have had episodes of epithelial rejection. Three had episodes of acute rejection that were managed by increasing systemic immunosuppression, and have resolved. Four patients have had chronic rejection, which has been treated by adjusting their systemic immunosuppression. In this study, 20 eyes (65.5 percent) out of 31 eyes underwent subsequent penetrating keratoplasty after keratolimbal allograft, which was successful in 14 eyes (70 percent)[14] and failed in 6 (30 percent). Twenty-six eyes (83.9 percent) presented with glaucoma. Four eyes had had a previous shunting procedure, and one had had a trabeculectomy before presentation.

After KLAL, 10 eyes (32.3 percent) had a subsequent tube shunt procedure because of uncontrolled intraocular pressure. Glaucoma is common in aniridia. In patients with limbal transplant and penetrating keratoplasty, the use of topical steroids further increases the intraocular pressure. Therefore, aniridic patients with severe glaucoma requiring more than two eyedrops for glaucoma treatment should undergo a tube shunt procedure before stem cell transplantation.[14,18] The

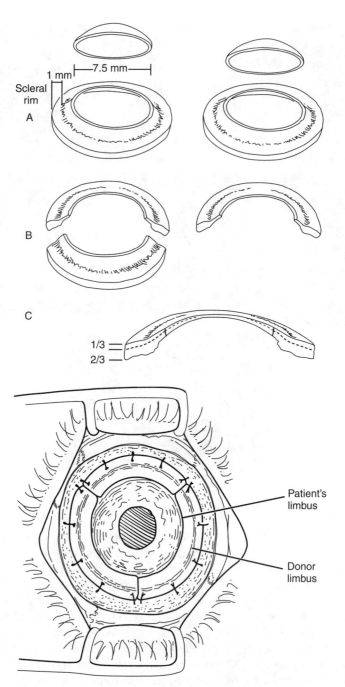

Figure 6.3 A color version of this figure may be viewed on the companion CD. Reprinted with permission of Springer Science and Business Media, from Edward J. Holland and Mark Mannis, *Ocular Surface Disease: Medical and Surgical Management*, 2002.

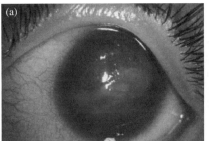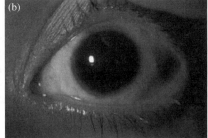

Figure 6.4 (a/b) A color version of this figure may be viewed on the companion CD. Reprinted with permission from personal library of Edward J. Holland, M.D.

Table 6.1 Immunosuppressive Regimen after Keratolimbal Allograft Transplantation

Agent	Dosage and Duration	Monitoring
Corticosteroids		
Topical	qid–qd, indefinitely	IOP, epithelial healing
Oral	1 mg/kg/day, taper over 6 months	BP, serum glucose, weight, gastritis, bone density, lipids
Cyclosporine A		
Topical	0.05%–2% bid–qid, indefinitely	Epithelial toxicity (vehicle)
Oral+	3 mg/kg/day, 12–18 months	Serum level 100–150 ng/dl, creatinine, BP, lipids, LFTs minerals (Mg), urinalysis, CBC q month
OR		
Tacrolimus+	1–4 mg bid, 12–18 months	Serum level 8–10 ng/ml first 3 months, then 5–8 ng/ml, creatinine, BP, lipids, LFTs minerals (Mg), urinalysis, CBC q month
Azathioprine*	100 mg/day, 12–18 months	CBC q month, chemistries, LFTs q 12 weeks
OR		
Mycophenolate*	500 mg bid, 12–18 months	CBC q month, chemistries LFTs q 12 weeks

* Only one of these two agents is used. + Only one of these two agents is used. IOP—intraocular pressure, BP—blood pressure, LFT—liver function test, CBC—complete blood count. Mg—Magnesium.

tube shunt procedure creates an artificial drainage pathway for intraocular fluid and helps in alleviating glaucoma.

Thus, according to Holland et al., keratolimbal allograft is effective in treating aniridic keratopathy. Patients receiving systemic immunosuppression have a significantly greater likelihood of achieving ocular surface stability. The patients with keratolimbal allograft should receive systemic immunosuppression with multidrug regime for 12 to 18 months after the procedure[14,18] (see Table 6.1). Keratolimbal allograft improves the success rate of subsequent penetrating keratoplasty.

ARTIFICIAL CORNEA

An eye that has had multiple corneal graft failure and cannot tolerate systemic immunosuppressive medication may benefit from an artificial cornea (kerato-prosthesis). An artificial cornea is a synthetic cornea offered to patients who are unlikely to be managed successfully by means of standard penetrating kerato-plasty. The complications associated with keratoprosthesis include glaucoma, corneal stromal meltdown, infection, endophthalmitis, retinal detachment, and retroprosthetic membrane formation.[19–21] Keratoprosthesis is thought to have a higher complication rate than conventional donor tissue grafts but has a promising role in the management of corneal blindness in patients with complex ocular disease and at higher risk of graft failure. The two commonly used artificial corneas are AlphaCor and Dohlman-Doane/Boston keratoprosthesis. AlphaCor is a flexible, one-piece synthetic cornea made of the hydrogel (2 hydroxy ethyl methacrylate/PHEMA).[22] The Dohlman-Doane keratoprosthesis is a rigid double-plated or collar-button shape made of polymethyl methacrylate (PMMA).[23] The successful use of the Boston keratoprosthesis in management of aniridic eyes has been reported recently.[24]

LENS PROBLEMS

Lens abnormalities in patients with aniridia include cataract, microphakia, and lens subluxation. Cortical, nuclear, and posterior subcapsular types of cataract are seen in patients with aniridia.[6] Patients may be myopic, emmetropic, or highly hyperopic. As the lens becomes cataractous or dislocates superiorly, a high degree of lenticular astigmatism is typical.[6]

Prevalence of Lens Problems

Cataract develops in 50 percent to 85 percent of patients with aniridia, usually during the first two decades of life.[6] Lens subluxation, also known as *ectopia lentis*, has been reported in ranges from 0 to 56 percent of patients with aniridia.[6,13,25,26] The diagnosis of the cataract can be made with the slit lamp examination. Sometimes, examination of the lens with the retinoscope and direct ophthalmo-scope may help in making the diagnosis.

Management of Lens Problems Associated with Aniridia

Cataract Management

In the initial stage of cataract when the vision loss is not significant, the use of corrective refractive glasses in the form of spectacles and contact lenses may improve the vision. However, when cataract extraction is required because of the inability to restore functional vision by optical means, it should be undertaken with awareness that the lenses of aniridic individuals may be poorly anchored, and some young aniridic patients have a thin and fragile anterior capsule.[27] In adults, both the intracapsular and the extracapsular technique have been employed, and the choice probably depends on the stability of the zonules,[6] the supporting system of the lens in the eye. If the zonules are stable, extracapsular cataract extraction (by phacoe-mulsification—use of ultrasound energy to break up and remove the cataract) technique is preferred as it is less traumatic to the corneal endothelium and gives a more stable and secure wound. Intracapsular cataract extraction, rarely performed these days, is done for severe zonular instability and lens subluxation. Vitreous humor can come forward as a complication of this procedure. Intracapsular cataract extraction involves removal of the entire lens and the capsule, while extracapsular extraction involves removal of the lens nucleus and cortex through an opening in the anterior capsule, leaving the capsular bag in place. Cataract extraction in children, rarely required, is probably best done by lensectomy technique, using an aspiration and cutting instrument.[6] Care should be taken to avoid tearing the anterior capsule during the cataract surgery. This could be achieved by using a highly retentive viscoelastic agent, injecting indocyanine green or trypan blue to stain the capsule, and making the capsulorhexis slightly smaller.[27]

Aniridic patients are operated on for subluxated lens if any of the following criteria are met:

- Best corrected visual acuity of less than 20/70
- Forward subluxation of lens to the anterior chamber
- Monocular diplopia
- Rapidly progressing posterior subluxation of the lens.[32]

The surgery for subluxated lenses includes lensectomy of ectopia lentis combined with anterior vitrectomy using a closed-system technique.[32] The closed-system technique maintains the anatomic relation of the eye, with no vitreous loss and no traction on the retina.[32]

Intraocular Lens. The majority of the lenses commonly used after cataract surgery are fabricated from either acrylic or silicone material (flexible) or polymethyl methacrylate (rigid). However, patients with aniridia have deficient irises, resulting in glare and photophobia. To overcome this disability, single-piece iris diaphragm intraocular lenses have been tried recently. This improves visual function by correcting the iris deficiency and restoring the phakic state at the same time. It consists of a full iris diaphragm surrounding a central optic. The commonly used iris diaphragm intraocular lens is the black diaphragm intraocular lens (Morcher type 67F and 67G) developed by Sundmacher et al.[28] The full iris diaphragm is about 10mm in diameter surrounding a central optic about 5mm in diameter. Reinhard et al. have conducted a study on 19 eyes from 14 patients with black diaphragm intraocular lens implant for congenital aniridia. In their study, 75 percent of the patients had improved visual acuity, and 80 percent had reduced glare after the procedure.[28]

The disadvantage with the use of black diaphragm intraocular lens is that the lens is rigid and brittle, making its manipulation during the surgery technically difficult, and requiring a larger incision due to the lens's relatively large size.[28] The two common postoperative complications seen are persistent intraocular inflammation and worsening glaucoma.[28] Therefore, patients should be carefully monitored after the black diaphragm intraocular lens implant.

Artificial Iris.   To overcome the drawback of the relatively large incision required by the iris-diaphragm intraocular lens, a system was designed in which the optic portion and the iris diaphragm are inserted separately. Volker Rash, from Germany, developed an endocapsular ring with iris diaphragm (Type 50C Morcher), which does not have an optical portion. It can be inserted through the same small incision as the foldable intraocular lens. The other endocapsular iris ring implant used is a single-fin 96G type developed by Rash and Rosenthal. These endocapsular rings are made of polymethyl methacrylate (PMMA) with an overall diameter of about 10.75 mm.[29] The endocapsular location of these implants avoids irritation to the ciliary body and angle structure, thereby minimizing postoperative inflammation.[29] The drawback of these implants is that they are brittle and susceptible to fracture during implantation.[29] Another disadvantage of prosthetic iris devices is the need for additional intraocular lenses to achieve optical correction in aphakia (patients without a lens due to prior cataract surgery where a lens was not placed in the eye).[30] Recently, Srinivasan et al. have conducted a retrospective study in five eyes of four patients with endocapsular iris reconstruction implants due to iris defects. According to their study, implantation of endocapsular iris reconstruction implants during cataract surgery appears to be a safe and effective technique in reducing glare disability and improving vision outcome.[29] Implantation of an artificial elastic iris-lens diaphragm following cataract surgery in patients with iris deficiency has also been reported in a recently conducted study to be effective in reducing glare disability and improving vision outcomes.[30] The latest design of an elastic artificial iris-lens diaphragm with a colored haptic— parts of the artificial lens that provide support and centration—is manufactured by photopolymerization of spatially linked polyoxypropylene.[30] The described model of artificial iris-lens diaphragm was implanted in 19 patients (20 eyes) with combined iris and lens pathology. Fifteen eyes (75 percent) experienced improvement in corrected visual activity. Glare and photophobia improved in all patients. One case of intraoperative vitreous hemorrhage and two cases of hyphema were reported, along with one postoperative instance of ciliochoroidal detachment. Chronic low-grade inflammation persisted in one eye, and intraocular pressure rise was reported in one eye. Documented cystoid macular edema occurred in one eye.[30]

Another implant used is the Ophtec model 311 iris construction lens. To date, 14 investigators at 11 sites have implanted over 140 of these devices; as of this writing it is expected to be submitted to the Food and Drug Administration for consideration. It is a single-piece implant made from clear and colored ultraviolet light–absorbing polymethyl methcrylate (PMMA). It is designed for implantation into aphakic and pseudophakic eyes (eyes that have had cataract extraction and placement of intraocular lens). This artificial iris lens is available in brown, blue, or green color. The clear central portion is available in powers of +10 to +30 diopters (in 0.5-diopter increments), or it can be ordered without power. The colored portion of the lens has a 9mm outer diameter and fixed 4mm inner diameter. One-year outcomes are now available for first 100 eyes with this implant. Among 100 eyes treated with this implant, 28 had congenital aniridia, 62 had traumatic injury, and 10 had surgical trauma. After the implant, 70 percent of the patient reports none to mild–photophobia, and 79 percent of patients report improvement in glare from mild to none. (Reference: Aniridia Insight Physicians and Researchers' Newsletter, Spring 2006).

COMPLICATIONS OF INTRAOCULAR SURGERY IN ANIRIDIA

Aniridic Fibrosis Syndrome

Aniridic patients with a history of previous intraocular surgery may develop aniridic fibrosis syndrome. The syndrome is characterized by the development of a progressive fibrotic membrane that appears to originate in the area of the rudimentary iris and can cause anterior displacement of the intraocular lens into the cornea.[31] The posterior extension of the membrane over the ciliary body may result in hypotony.[31] The risk of aniridic fibrosis syndrome increases with increasing intraocular hardware and procedures.[31] Recognition of the signs of aniridic fibrosis syndrome should trigger careful monitoring that includes serial A-scan measurement or ultrasonic biomicroscopy (see Table 6.2). If progression is noted, early surgical intervention, including explantation of the intraocular lens and/or artificial iris, is strongly indicated.[31] Early surgical intervention can prevent the complications associated with posterior and anterior extension of the fibrosis.[31]

SUMMARY

The corneal and lens problems seen in aniridia usually progresses with age. The main corneal problems seen in aniridia are the abnormalities of corneal epithelium

Table 6.2 Signs of Aniridic Fibrosis Syndrome

1	Retrolenticular fibrotic membrane
2	Retrocorneal fibrotic membrane
3	Forward displacement of intraocular lens
4	Hypotony (extension of fibrotic membrane over ciliary body)
5	Endothelial decompensation
6	Tractional retinal detachment

and subsequent progressive opacification of cornea from limbal stem cell deficiency. Other associated conditions include dry eyes, thickened central cornea, Peter's anomaly, and microcornea. The main lens-related problem is the development of cataract.

Management of aniridia is a constant challenge because of its complex nature, panocular manifestations, and progressive course. Keratolimbal allograft technique by Holland et al. for the management of aniridic keratopathy is a significant achievement. The artificial iris and intraocular lens developed in the last decade have a promising role in management of glare and photophobia. Given that PAX6 gene mutations have been found in approximately 80 percent of those tested for aniridia (both familial and sporadic),[33] development of a successful gene therapy for PAX6 mutation could play a vital role in the future in the management of aniridic keratopathy.

Notes

1. Schermer, A., Galvin, S., et al. (1986). Differentiation-related expression of a major 64K corneal keratin *in vivo* and in culture suggests limbal location of corneal eoithelium stem cells. *Journal of Cell Biology, 103,* 49–62.
2. Cotsarelis, G., Cheng, S. Z., et al. (1989). Existence of slow-cycling limbal epithelial basal cells that can be preferentially stimulated to proliferate: Implications on epithelial stem cells. *Cell, 57,* 201–209.
3. Thoft, R. A., & Friend, J. (1983). The X,Y, Z hypothesis of corneal epithelial maintenance. *Investigative Ophthalmology & Visual Science, 24,* 1442–1443.
4. Buck, R. C. (1985). Measurement of centripetal migration of normal corneal epithelial cells in the mouse. *Investigative Ophthalmology & Visual Science, 26,* 1296–1299.
5. Mackman, G., Brightbill, F. S., et al. (1979). Corneal changes in aniridia. *American Journal of Ophthalmology, 87,* 497–502.
6. Nelson, L. B., Spaeth, G. L., et al. (1984). Aniridia; a review. *Survey of Ophthalmology, 28,* 621–642.
7. Nishida, K., Kinoshita, S., et al. (1995). Ocular surface abnormalities in aniridia. *American Journal of Ophthalmology, 120,* 368–375.
8. Ramaesh, K., Ramaesh, T., et al. (2005). Evolving concepts on the pathogenic mechanisms of aniridia related keratopathy. *The International Journal of Biochemistry and Cell Biology, 37,* 547–557.
9. Ramesh, T., Collinson, J. M., et al. (2003). Corneal abnormalities in PAX6 small eye mice mimic human aniridia-related keratopathy. *Investigative Ophthalmology & Visual Science, 44,* 1871–1878.
10. Jastaneiah, S., & Al- Rajhi, A. A. (2005), Association of aniridia and dry eyes. *Ophthalmology, 112,* 1535–1540.
11. Mayer, U. M. (1992). Peters' anomaly and combination with other malformations (series of 16 patients). *Ophthalmic Pediatric Genetics, 13,* 131–5.
12. Brandt, J. D., Casuso, L. A., et al. (2004). Markedly increased central corneal thickness: An unrecognized finding in congenital aniridia. *American Journal of Ophthalmology, 137,* 348–350.

13. David, R., Macbeath, L., et al. (1978). Aniridia associated with microcornea and subluxated lens. *British Journal of Ophthalmology, 62*, 118–121.

14. Holland, E. J., Djalilian, , A. R., et al. (2003). Management of aniridic keratopathy with keratolimbal allograft: A limbal stem cell transplantation technique. *Ophthalmology, 110*, 125–130.

15. Gomes, J. A. P., Eagle, R. C., et al. (1996). Recurrent keratopathy after penetrating keratoplasty for aniridia. *Cornea, 15*, 457–462.

16. Holland, E. J., & Schwartz, G. S. (1996). The evolution of epithelial transplantation for severe ocular surface disease and a proposed classification system. *Cornea, 15*, 549–566.

17. Tseng, S. C. G., Prabhasawant, P., et al. (1998). Amniotic membrane transplantation with or without limbal allografts for corneal surface reconstruction in patients with limbal stem cell deficiency. *Archives of Ophthalmology, 116*, 431–441.

18. Kim, J. Y., Djalilian, A. R., et al. (2003). Ocular surface reconstruction: Limbal stem cell transplantation. *Ophthalmology Clinics North America, 16*, 67–77.

19. Hicks, C. R., Crawford, G. J., et al. (2003). Corneal replacement using a synthetic hydrogel cornea, AlphaCor device: Preliminary outcome and complications. *Eye, 17*, 385–392.

20. Ma, J. J. K., Graney, J. M., et al. (2005). Repeat penetrating keratoplasty versus the Boston keratoprosthesis in graft failure. *International Ophthalmology Clinics, 45*, 49–59.

21. Sarac, I. O., Akpek, E. K., et al. (2005). Current concepts and techniques in keratoprosthesis. *Current Opinion in Ophthalmology, 16*, 246–250.

22. Hicks, Crawford (2003), 385–392.

23. Doane, M. G., Dohlman, C. H., et al. (1996). Fabrication of keratoprosthesis. *Cornea, 15*, 179–184.

24. Khan, B. F., Dagher, M. H., et al. (2006). Herpetic keratitis and aniridia: Boston keratoprosthesis. Presented at the Association for Research in Vision and Ophthalmology 2006 annual conference.

25. Shaw, M. W., Falls, H. F., Neel, J. V. (1960). Congenital aniridia. *American Journal of Human Genetics, 12*, 389–415.

26. Callahan, A. (1949). Aniridia with ectopia lentis and secondary glaucoma: Genetic, pathologic and surgical considerations. *American Journal of Ophthalmology, 28*, 39–47.

27. Schneider, S., Osher, R. H., et al. (2003). Thinning of the anterior capsule associated with congenital aniridia. *Journal of Cataract Refractive Surgery, 29*, 523–525.

28. Reinhard, T., & Engelhardt, S. (2000). Black diaphragm aniridia intraocular lens for congenital aniridia: Long-term follow-up. *Journal of Cataract Refractive Surgery, 26*, 375–381.

29. Srinivasan, S., Yuen, C., et al. (2006). Endocapsular iris reconstruction implants for acquired iris defects: A clinical study. *Eye, 9*, 1–5.

30. Pozdeyeva, N. A., & Pashtayev, N. P. (2005). Artificial iris-lens diaphragm in reconstructive surgery for aniridia and aphakia. *Journal of Cataract and Refractive Surgery, 31*, 1750–1759.

31. Tsai, J. H., Freeman, J. M., et al. (2005). A progressive anterior fibrosis syndrome in patients with postsurgical congenital aniridia. *American Journal of Ophthalmology, 140*, 1075–1107.

32. Halpert, M., Benezra, D., et al. (1996). Surgery of the hereditary subluxated lens in children. *Ophthalmology, 103*, 681–686.
33. Axton, R., Hanson, I., et al. (1997). The incidence of PAX6 mutation in patients with simple aniridia: An evaluation of mutation detection in 12 cases. *Journal of Medical Genetics, 34*, 279–286.

7

Low Vision and Aniridia

JENNIFER K. BULMANN

Aniridia affects many visual aspects of one's life. This chapter will highlight many of these effects. Functional changes that occur due to aniridia will be discussed. Once the patient's vision is assessed and goals are established with a thorough eye examination, numerous avenues can be taken to ensure the support of all the patient's health care providers. Referrals can be made to appropriate professionals to ensure full understanding and management of the ocular condition.

FUNCTIONAL VISION CHANGES AND ANIRIDIA

Visual Acuity

Visual acuity is the measurement used to determine vision levels. Normal vision is 20/20, which means that what a normal person sees at 20 feet, the patient sees at 20 feet. If their vision is 20/40, they would need to be at a distance of 20 feet to see what someone with normal vision can see at 40 feet.

The decrease in visual acuity in those with aniridia usually ranges from under 20/60 to as low as approximately 20/400. This is due to the lack of development of the macular area, or fovea. The fovea is responsible for our clearest, most precise vision.

Those with visual acuity of 20/200 or worse that is best corrected while wearing spectacles or contact lenses in the better-seeing eye are considered legally blind. While most people who suffer from aniridia are not legally blind, they are visual impaired. Visual impairment is defined as visual acuity of 20/70 in the better-seeing eye when optimally corrected with glasses or contact lenses. The designation of "visual impairment" also has a functionality factor. If a person has a reduction in the ability of the eye or the visual system to perform to a normal ability, he/she is considered visually impaired.

95

Visual Field

Visual field is the measurement of peripheral vision. Those with aniridia may have decreased peripheral vision. This is not directly due to aniridia, but rather to glaucoma, which may develop due to structural changes in the eye. Glaucoma is explained in detail in the glaucoma chapter of this book. If a patient has adequate visual acuity, but has a decreased visual field of 20 degrees or less at its widest diameter, he or she is considered legally blind.

Contrast/Glare/Photophobia

Most aniridia patients experience extreme light sensitivity (photophobia). This is because the enlarged pupil allows more light to enter the eye. The pupil is actually a hole that allows light to be viewed on the retina. The amount of light entering the eye is determined by the muscles in the colored part of the eye (iris). In aniridia, the iris, which typically blocks much of the light entering the eye, is not fully developed.

Because of the extra light entering the eye, patients may notice glare, such as "halos" around lights, which can interfere with the sharpness of the image. When the pupils are large in those with aniridia, they may notice that the contrast between light colors and dark colors may be more difficult to see.

Oculomotor Symptoms — Strabismus/Nystagmus

Some patients with aniridia may have an eye that turns inward or outward (strabismus). This eye turn is due to the macular area's being unable to focus clearly. This occurs because the macular area is underdeveloped in those with aniridia. When the macula is unable to see clearly, the eyes tend to have a repetitive, involuntary swinging motion left and right (nystagmus). These two findings will be present early in life, and may help aid in a diagnosis.

SIGHT EVALUATION/TESTING MODIFICATIONS

Correction of Refractive Error

Refractive error is the term used when someone needs glasses for distant and/or close activities. Patients with aniridia may have farsightedness (hyperopia), nearsightedness (myopia), or astigmatism, just like anyone else. There is no predetermination for any one type of refractive error.

Spectacles can be prescribed for those who have a refractive error. It is recommended that impact-resistant (polycarbonate) lenses be prescribed. Polycarbonate lenses are safety lenses that are used for children and those with decreased vision due to eye diseases or trauma.

Contact lenses can also be worn in those with aniridia, as long as the front, clear surface of the eye (cornea) is healthy. Research has stimulated controversy about

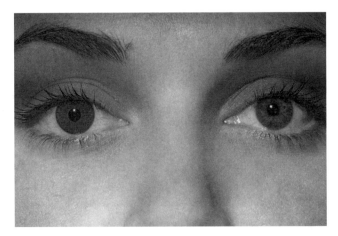

Figure 7.1 Right eye of a patient with an opaque contact lens in place.
Photos by: Phil Ridings, Southern College of Optometry.

using contact lenses to decrease the amount of nystagmus. Some report that wearing contact lenses decreases the stimulation to the brain, thus decreasing the nystagmus. Others report that wearing contact lenses increases the patient's awareness of the involuntary eye movements.

Specialty contact lenses have been determined to be useful in those with aniridia. Because of their large pupils and decreased size of their irises, painted contact lenses are beneficial (such contact lenses are artificially pigmented irises and artificially darkened pupils). Because the contact lenses are darkened, the amount of light entering the eye is decreased. These lenses will primarily reduce complaints of photophobia, glare, and contrast. These lenses will not necessarily improve visual acuity more than normal spectacle lenses (see Figure 7.1).

Management of Oculomotor Issues

Nystagmus (involuntary oscillating eye movement) develops at a very young age in those with aniridia. If it is present since birth, it is called *congenital nystagmus.* Patients who have this condition may have a "null point," or an ability to point their eyes a certain direction to decrease the amount of involuntary eye movements. A prism can be introduced in front of the eyes to help decrease the amount of a head tilt or head turn. Prisms in glasses move the image that is seen to a different position, allowing patients to not have to tilt or turn their heads as much to decrease the amount of nystagmus.

Vision therapy is an option for those who have a strabismus, or eye turn due to muscle weakness. Vision therapy can help develop the eye muscles, which in turn would improve eye alignment. A workup can be done by a specially trained optometrist to determine what course of action should be taken in this area.

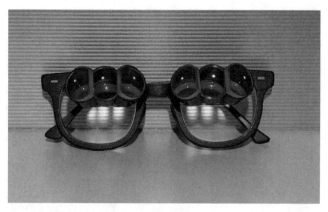

Figure 7.2 Example of a field expander.
Photos by: Phil Ridings, Southern College of Optometry.

Management of Visual Field Issues

When a patient with aniridia is diagnosed with glaucoma, the doctor will make every effort to lower the pressure in the eye so as to maintain the peripheral vision. If the visual field is compromised, patients will complain of running into walls, being unable to see where they are walking, hitting their heads, or having to turn their heads to see things around them, just to name a few of the related problems. Visual field testing will help determine the amount of their peripheral field loss.

If their peripheral vision is significantly decreased, field expanders may be recommended. These devices will increase a person's degree of side vision. Field expanders contain prism lenses, which can move objects from the unseeing area into the seeing area of the retina (see Figure 7.2).

Canes may be used to help patients with decreased peripheral vision to "feel" the area to the sides and in front of where they are walking. Mobility training can help those patients adjust to this kind of walking, as it is tedious and difficult for the novice.

LOW VISION DEVICE EVALUATION

Magnification for Near Activities

Most aniridia patients have difficulty with near activities. These activities include such things as reading newspapers, books, menus, price tags, medicine bottles, etc. There are numerous options to better their vision for closeup work. Once a distance prescription is determined and finalized, the near tasks can be addressed.

Many times a simple higher-power aid for near activities can be prescribed. Aniridia patients are highly successful with higher-powered bifocals for reading. When a high-power aid is recommended, the patients need to realize that they may need to hold their reading material a little bit closer than normal.

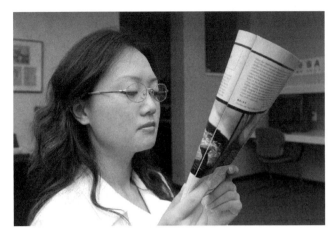

Figure 7.3 A patient wearing a pair of bifocals with a high power lens for near. Notice the closer working distance in order to view the magazine clearly.
Photos by: Phil Ridings, Southern College of Optometry.

They may notice that the working distance is a little uncomfortable at first; however, the print will appear larger and therefore clearer with the increase in power (see Figure 7.3).

At times, a patient may want to wear reading-only glasses. Half-eye glasses with a prism work well for people who enjoy reading for extended periods of time. The appearance of the glasses is similar to that of small reading glasses that can be purchased over the counter; however, the power of the spectacles is much stronger. The prism in the glasses helps to relax the eyes when reading (see Figure 7.4).

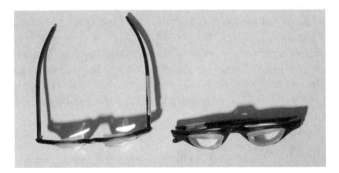

Figure 7.4 Two pair of prism half-eye glasses. Notice the thickness close to where the glasses sit on the nose. They contain prism, which allows the patient's eyes to relax while reading.
Photos by: Phil Ridings, Southern College of Optometry.

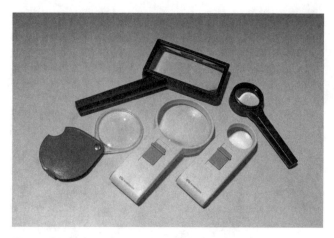

Figure 7.5 Hand held magnifiers pictured. Both the lighted and non-lighted versions are shown.
Photos by: Phil Ridings, Southern College of Optometry.

Another option is to use a handheld magnifier. There are many different powers available. Some may only need lower-powered/larger magnifiers, while others may need a higher-powered/smaller magnifier. With the higher-powered handheld magnifier, the area to view through becomes smaller, but the images through the magnifier will be larger. There are lighted and non-lighted models. The lighted magnifiers work extremely well in a dark restaurant or at the theater, for example. There are also pocket-sized magnifiers. These can be conveniently carried in a small bag or suit-jacket pocket (see Figure 7.5).

Stand magnifiers also exist, with or without a light. Stand magnifiers have a set focusing distance, so they are placed directly onto the page. The page *and* magnifier are moved closer or farther from one's eye to view the reading material. These work well for those with shaky hands, such as someone with Parkinson's disease. Remember, the stronger the power, the smaller the device. It also means a smaller lens to look through compared to the lower-powered magnifiers (see Figures 7.6 and 7.7).

It is also important to incorporate lighting into reading tasks. It must be decided whether having a bright light over the shoulder will help, or conversely, would only increase the glare. Lights come in many different forms. Gooseneck lighting works well for near tasks (see Figure 7.8). Regular overhead lights work well for other nonspecific tasks.

Magnification for Distance Activities

Most aniridia patients will need help in the distance as well. Although a precise determination of their prescription, called *refraction*, is imperative, vision may not be adequate enough to see finer details such as street signs or stoplights.

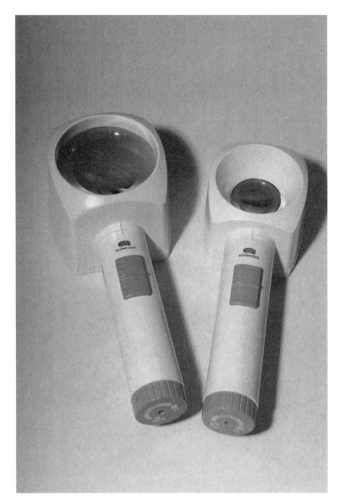

Figure 7.6 Lighted stand magnifiers.
Photos by: Phil Ridings, Southern College of Optometry.

For those with aniridia who are in the classroom, numerous devices are available. Viewing the blackboard or overheads may be difficult, as well as PowerPoint presentations that are projected at the front of the room. Monocular telescopes are available to place in front of the better-seeing eye for viewing words or diagrams. They can be handheld to be placed in front of spectacles to spot-check, or they can be mounted into a pair of glasses (see Figure 7.9). If the vision in each eye individually is approximately the same, binocular telescopes can be prescribed (see Figure 7.10). Telescopes that can be adjusted to have variable focus points are usually recommended so that vision is clear at numerous distances, depending on the task at hand.

Many states allow bioptic telescope driving. Bioptics are telescopes that are mounted into the upper position in a pair of spectacles (see Figure 7.11). There are

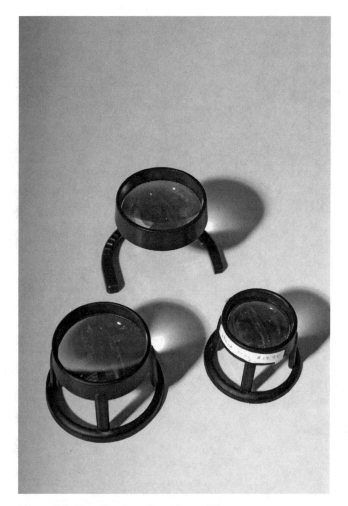

Figure 7.7 Non-illuminated stand magnifiers.
Photos by: Phil Ridings, Southern College of Optometry.

many different sizes and powers of telescopes that can be used and recommended. States that allow bioptic driving have laws that vary from state to state based on visual acuity and peripheral vision. It is important to note that if a patient resides in a state that allows bioptic driving and they have a driver's license, they are allowed to drive in any other state, even if that state doesn't allow their licensed drivers to do so.

A thorough examination to determine eligibility should be performed by an optometrist specializing in the fitting of bioptics. Once the patient's eligibility is determined, each state has requirements for driver's education. (See the state's Department of Motor Vehicles for details.)

Other distance tasks may be addressed with low-vision devices. Patients may want to enjoy television, sports games, or theater or movies. Television and sports glasses are available to be used for such events. They are similar to the binocular telescopes,

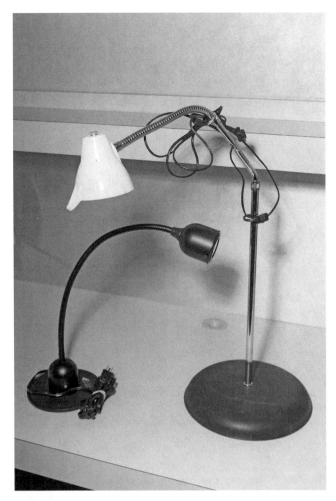

Figure 7.8 Gooseneck lamps. These can be placed on a desk or over the shoulder of the patient.
Photos by: Phil Ridings, Southern College of Optometry.

but are less expensive and lighter in weight when worn (see Figure 7.12). These devices can also be used for reading music while playing an instrument. These are capable of having a shorter working distance than the telescopes used in the class-room. They allow the intermediate distance to be addressed.

Electronic Magnification

There are times when magnifiers, reading glasses, bifocals, and/or telescopes are not adequate due to significant vision loss or comfort factors. When one needs higher powers at near viewing, or needs increased comfort, closed circuit televisions (CCTVs) make for easier reading and other near-at-hand tasks.

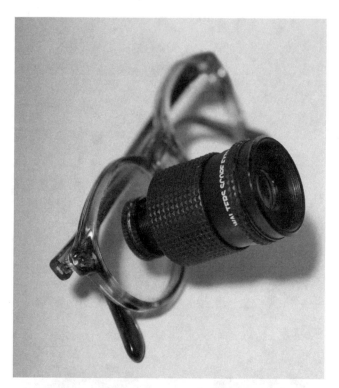

Figure 7.9 Monocular telescope mounted into a pair of glasses in the "straight ahead" position. These work well for classroom work. Photos by: Phil Ridings, Southern College of Optometry.

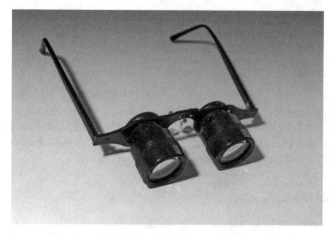

Figure 7.10 Sport glasses. These are used for distance activities including sporting events or the theater.
Photos by: Phil Ridings, Southern College of Optometry.

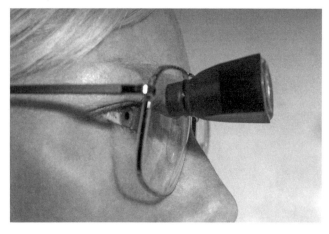

Figure 7.11 Telescope used for driving in states that allow. Also known as a bi-optic. Notice the upper position of the telescope. This is to view straight ahead for driving and to lean head down in order to spot street signs.
Photos by: Phil Ridings, Southern College of Optometry.

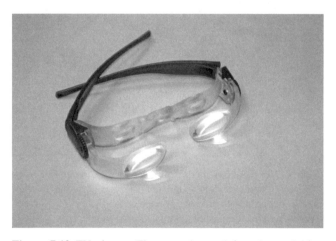

Figure 7.12 TV glasses. These can be used for other activities such as reading music on a piano.
Photos by: Phil Ridings, Southern College of Optometry.

CCTVs come in different forms. There are desktop models that are the approximate size of a desktop computer. There is a screen at eye level and a moving platform below. The platform moves for ease of reading. There is a built-in camera that transfers the material on the platform to the screen above. Magnification can reach up to nearly 50 times as large as normal newspaper print. Not only is reading facilitated, but writing, painting, and arts and crafts as well (see Figure 7.13).

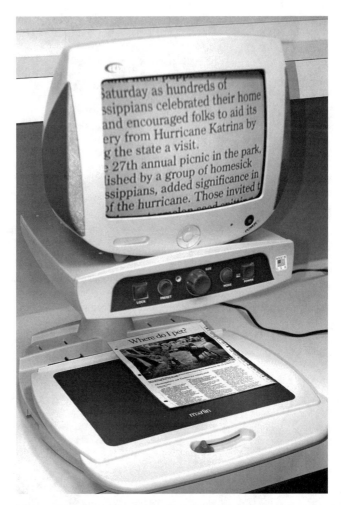

Figure 7.13 Desktop model of the Closed Circuit Television (CCTV). These are bulky and not as portable. Able to view newspaper print with ease in this photo.
Photos by: Phil Ridings, Southern College of Optometry.

If patients want to take the CCTV with them, portable models are available. They look like a mouse used with a computer. Within the "mouse" is a camera. The device hooks into any television. The larger the television, the larger the print appears on the TV screens. A patient is able to write with the portable CCTV as long as the device is angled so as to watch the pen/pencil in the television (see Figure 7.14).

Activities of Daily Living

Once the determination of a spectacle prescription, near-device evaluation, and distance-device evaluation takes place, the optometrist will discuss the patient's

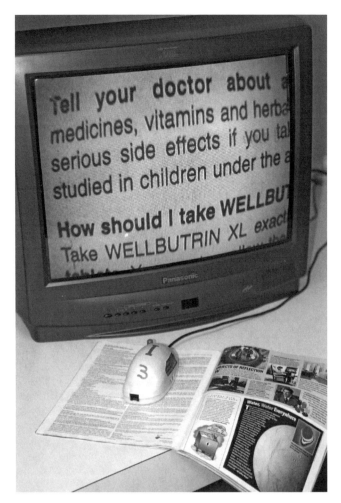

Figure 7.14 Portable CCTV. This has the appearance of a computer mouse. These are portable. Able to view drug advertisement with ease in this photo.
Photos by: Phil Ridings, Southern College of Optometry.

needs in daily living activities. Activities of daily living (ADLs) include but are not limited to cooking using a stove, microwave, and oven; laundry; dishes; personal grooming; and other household chores. Bump dots or fluorescent paint can be placed on buttons and knobs to help the person tell temperature and see if controls are on or off. High-contrast measuring cups and spoons can be used to help in the kitchen as well (e.g., black measuring cups used to measure flour or sugar). Magnifying mirrors can help with personal grooming and makeup application. Talking watches or watches with large numbered faces can be recommended. These are just a few examples of the devices available (see Figure 7.15).

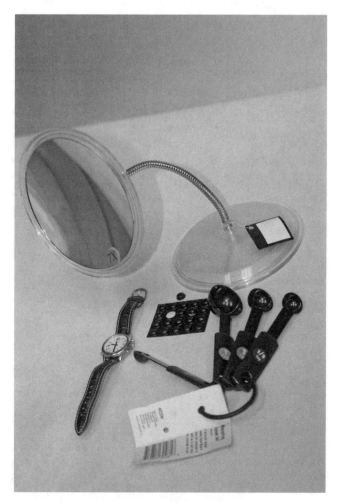

Figure 7.15 Some tools to help make things easier: a magnified mirror, talking watch, and larger print measuring spoons.
Photos by: Phil Ridings, Southern College of Optometry.

MULTIDISCIPLINARY TEAM APPROACH

Treating low vision is not accomplished just by the doctor prescribing the devices. Once devices are recommended, other disciplines in the rehabilitative services are utilized.

ADL instructors work with patients to teach them skills they needed to cope with everyday activities. Orientation and mobility (O&M) specialists will also be used. O&M instructors work with patients who have difficulty getting around. They concentrate on how independent movement plays a role in activities. They teach patients how to move from place to place confidently, comfortably, and safely. Many instructors work with loss of depth perception, loss of contrast, loss of color, and loss of visual field (which is common in those with advanced glaucoma). If a patient is legally blind, white-cane training is included in this specialty.

Low-vision therapists use the recommendations by the eye care specialist to work with the patient. They continue to work on the visual function of the aniridia patients, teaching and training them to use spectacles—reading only, distance only, or bifocal—and other near and distance devices efficiently. They also teach them how to modify their environment (lighting, seating) to maximize their visual potential. Part of low-vision therapists' work is counseling family members in the use of devices and how to help aniridia sufferers.

The multidisciplinary team will meet many times to make sure that the patient is doing well and meeting goals in all areas of low vision. This helps to decrease any redundancy or weaknesses in training that might take place.

PROFESSIONALS INVOLVED IN LOW-VISION REHABILITATION

Many professionals are involved in the low-vision rehabilitation process. Once the diagnosis of aniridia is established, it is important to make sure the different specialty areas are informed.

The primary care doctor needs to be made aware of the patient's problem with vision, so as to be able to follow any possible systemic problems as well. Co-management with an ophthalmologist is important if the diagnosis of glaucoma is determined. Possible surgical intervention in the future may be needed. Occupational therapists (OTs) and physical therapists (PTs) may work with the patient to improve their quality of life. They will stress independent living skills.

Those with aniridia may want to discuss with psychologists, sociologists, or counselors issues pertaining to their vision loss. Dealing with vision loss is a very difficult personal issue, and many times it helps to talk about it. Professionals who are trained in the acknowledgment and acceptance of vision loss can help deal with psychosocial issues pertaining to aniridia. They are also a great resource for support groups that enable patients to talk to others with similar conditions.

Aniridia has been found to be genetically linked. If a patient is considering having children, a geneticist can discuss the genetic components of the disease.

While aniridia is a vision-threatening disease, many devices are available to aid in near and distance tasks, activities of daily living, and orientation and mobility training. The multidisciplinary team approach assures all the needs of patients with aniridia are addressed.

Patients with aniridia have to know that when the words "nothing else can be done, you just have to deal with this" are spoken, it is time to make an appointment with an eye care professional who specializes in the area of low vision. These professionals can help improve the functionality of the eyesight of those with vision loss, and direct them to appropriate support groups.

8

Psychological Support

MARK PISHOTTA AND ALISON KRANGEL

Stress is an everyday experience that no one is exempt from experiencing, whether the stressor is positive or negative. Combine that reality with a medical condition, and there is a noticeable increase in the stress level that can easily become overwhelming.

Like other diagnoses, aniridia has an impact on those living with the condition and their families. One of the reasons this condition is so complex is the lack of knowledge about it in both the public and medical communities. Too often people respond with a "What?" when they hear the word *aniridia*, and that leaves the families to be the educators, when they are the ones who still need to be educated.

Their frustration can easily build. There is frustration with the diagnosis, with the life changes, and with the frustration itself. Without recognition or acceptance of this frustration, and an appropriate outlet to help ease the situation, negative effects are likely. It is vital for those touched by aniridia to prepare for the inevitable stress. Parents must identify and accept themselves as the supporting structures of their families. If they are weakened, they will be less likely to support their children. Individuals with aniridia have enough barriers to overcome and must learn to prevent future obstacles such as stress from affecting their lives. Although stress is unavoidable, it is at times preventable and, most often, manageable.

By and large, there are three types of stress: acute, episodic, and chronic. *Acute stress* is defined as short-term stress that does not result in any permanent damage. One can describe this as the daily stress that can be lived with and is experienced by all individuals (such as taking tests and driving in heavy traffic). The second stress, *episodic stress*, is more intense because it is the frequent suffering of acute stress. The sufferer views life as chaotic and constantly in crisis, epitomized by the expression "if something can go wrong, it will." Not all individuals are exposed to this type of stress. Finally, *chronic stress* is the result of unrelenting demands and pressure; it often results in long-term effects. Examples include poverty, dysfunctional home life, and, of course, illnesses. Individuals with aniridia definitely fall into this category, and, as a result, are prone to at least two and possibly all three types of stress.

In school, a child with aniridia might feel acute stress when it is his turn to read out loud in class. As he picks up his book and puts his nose right up to the page, he will feel his classmates staring straight at him, whether in actuality or only in his imagination. He may feel embarrassed because, in his mind, his peers see him as different and weird. He will begin to feel self-conscious, his heartbeat will speed up, and he will begin to sweat.

An individual with aniridia may experience episodic stress each time she goes to an eye doctor appointment. Her thought process might be, "I know he is going to find something wrong with my eyes. My pressure will probably be too high. What if my vision has gotten worse? What if he tells me I need surgery? Nothing else has been going right this week, why should this be any different?"

Chronic stress will always afflict, not only persons with aniridia, but also parents of children with aniridia. Parents are always thinking about their children and how to make life better for them. They worry that their child is not getting the help he needs in school or is not fitting in with his peer group. They are always thinking about the upcoming doctor's appointments or what the future has in store for their child. These thoughts and feelings are so ingrained in their minds that they come as naturally as brushing their teeth or eating dinner.

There are two other categories of stress: external and internal. External stress is caused by forces outside an individual's control and is viewed as a natural part of life. Examples include accidents, weddings, and illnesses such as aniridia. Internal stress, on the other hand, is caused by an irrational cognitive thought process. This usually follows the external stress and serves to escalate the perception of stress.

It is important to identify internal stress. Aniridia patients and their families suffer from the external stress of the diagnosis and all the hardships the disease brings. However, if patients or families adopt the idea that aniridia is ruining their lives, they have added an internal stressor. External stress cannot be controlled by the individual, but internal stress can be. The challenge is to help families and individuals with aniridia realize that, while aniridia does complicate life, they have to remember that "difficult" does not equal "impossible."

It is in our best interests to deter irrational negative thoughts to avoid an overload of stress. One way to combat such thoughts is to use the *ABC model*, which is derived from a cognitive theory used predominately when dealing with anger.[1] The model suggests that all people experience an activating event or stressor (external stress)—the "A." From there, people develop beliefs (internal stress)—the "B"—which results in consequences or negative feelings—the "C."

The goal of the model would be to challenge the beliefs (B) by creating a different thought process—the "D." This would lead to an alternative effect or new way of perceiving the original problem—the "E."

Below are two examples that illustrate the model. The first example shows the model in its general form; the second adapts the model to those with aniridia.

Example 1

- A Activating event (external stressor)
- B Beliefs (internal stressor)

- C Consequences or feelings
- D Different way of thinking
- E Alternative effects or new ways of viewing the original problem

Example 2

- A Family or person receives diagnosis of aniridia (external stressor)
- B Original thought becomes "Life is ruined." (internal stressor)
- C Negative feelings such as depression develop
- D New thought becomes "This will be difficult, but I will manage"
- E New outlook becomes "Life has challenges, but it is still good"

It is important to recognize the various sources of stress. To simplify its origins, stress has been arranged here into four separate categories: personal and social, marital, vocational, and financial. These four groups serve to cover the major domains of a person's life.

Personal and Social

- Ill health of self and family
- Time pressure
- Unrealistic expectations
- Lack of goals and direction
- Lower self-esteem
- Increased self-doubt
- Hindered social life
- Difficulty dating
- Lack of physician awareness
- Misdiagnosis
- Physicians who discourage asking questions
- Increase in declining health of self

Marital

- Expectations not met
- Needs not satisfied
- Issues with communication
- Difficulty with role definition
- Lack of time devoted to spouse and/or family
- Separation or divorce
- Blaming self or spouse for disability/diagnosis
- Feeling unable to meet needs of disability/diagnosis
- Losing additional time due to doctor's appointments, treatments, or therapies
- High percentage of divorce

- Worry about children inheriting aniridia
- Living in denial

Vocational

- Employment dissatisfaction
- Feeling overworked and/or under appreciated
- Increased time spent at work
- Taking work home
- Misperception based on appearance (i.e., droopy eyes perceived as substance use)
- Stares from people because something is held too close to one's eyes
- Lack of transportation
- Difficulty meeting needs to complete work
- Fear of disrupting work environment or creating an inconvenience to others

Financial

- Failing to evaluate needs versus wants
- Poor prioritizing of funds
- Failing to create a strategy to cope
- Costs of medications, transplants, surgeries, transportation
- Lack of employment opportunities
- Time off from work
- Health insurance

In order for individuals to change, they must determine whether or not they identify a need to change. To do this, people engage in what research psychologist James Prochaska terms the *stages of change*[2]. In this model there are six stages: precontemplation, contemplation, preparation, action, maintenance, and relapse. In the first stage, precontemplation, the individual is not aware that there is a problem, or does not consider the situation important. This thought continues into the contemplation stage because the person is not seriously thinking about altering a particular behavior or thought, but they are thinking about the potential of changing. Not until the third stage, preparation, do they seriously consider their options and plan to change. The individual prepares herself or himself physically, intellectually, emotionally, and spiritually for change. By the action stage, the individual takes specific steps toward changing behaviors relative to the problem. In the maintenance stage, the individual works to sustain changes until they become customary. He or she consistently follows through on strategies to control stress, and adopts a proactive position by anticipating future obstacles. In the final stage, relapse, the person ceases to progress towards change either because they are not interested or are less concerned about maintaining the change.

Below is an example of how the stages of change could look in relation to stress.

Precontemplation: Person thinks, "I don't get bothered by stress."
Contemplation: Person's thought becomes, "So what if I get stressed, everyone gets stressed. It's no big deal, right?"
Preparation: Person develops new thought process: "Maybe I will research some stress-management techniques on the internet."
Action: Individual researches stress-management techniques and applies some of them.
Maintenance: Person continues to apply stress-management techniques.
Relapse: Person discontinues stress-management techniques.

Here is the thought process of a teenaged aniridia patient who is at the legal driving age.

Precontemplation: "I don't care that I can't drive."
Contemplation: "So what if I can't drive, it's easier to get chauffeured around anyway, right?"
Preparation: "Maybe I will research some stress-management techniques on the internet."
Action: "I think it might help if I take a walk when I start to feel angry about not being able to drive. Then, when I am calmer, I can write down my real feelings."
Maintenance: "I have been walking and writing in my journal for a month now, and I feel better."
Relapse: Hasn't written anything in a while.

It is important for individuals to evaluate where they see themselves in relation to change. If they have not identified a need themselves, or others have not mentioned it to them, there is little likelihood that anything will be altered. However, if the individual is mindful, either by their own account or due to the influence of others, it is likelier that they will change.

When stress occurs in minimal amounts, the effects are less noticeable; however, when the amount of stress intensifies, so do the effects. Below is a list of some effects of stress: physical, psychological and emotional, and social.

Physical Effects

- Tension or migraine headaches
- Irritable bowel, upset stomach, constipation, diarrhea
- Muscle tension, back and neck pain
- Fatigue
- Sleep disturbance
- High blood pressure, chest pain

- Skin problems
- Jaw pain (from clenching the jaw)
- Reproductive problems
- Immune system suppression

Psychological and Emotional Effects

- Nervousness or anxiety
- Feelings of depression or moodiness
- Irritability or frustration
- Lack of concentration
- Feeling out of control
- Phobias
- Overreaction

Social Effects

- Increased arguments
- Overreactions
- Conflict with others (family, peers or coworkers/employees)
- Loss of control with family or peers
- Frequent job changes
- Domestic or workplace violence
- Isolation from social activities
- Road rage

When the stress remains constant and relief is not sought, the individual is at risk for possible long-term effects listed below.

Possible Long-Term Effects

- Obesity
- Heart disease
- Diabetes
- Cancer
- Depression
- Posttraumatic Stress Disorder (PTSD) symptoms
- Anorexia nervosa or malnutrition
- Obsessive compulsive or anxiety disorder
- Substance abuse

Now that we understand what stress is and what it can do, the question becomes, How can one prevent stress from negatively impacting one's life? The good news is that there is a variety of techniques people can use. Picking the most appropriate one depends on the individual. Below are some helpful techniques one can use to reduce stress.

- Exercise
- Spirituality
- Journaling
- Deep breathing
- Progressive relaxation
- Mental imagery
- Create your own (music, reading, hobbies)

Exercising allows one's body to experience a physical release. It improves the immune system, so it is better able to defend against illness.

Spirituality is helpful because some people take comfort in the thought that Someone is looking after them. Think of the comfort a children receive knowing their parents will take care of them. Believing in a higher power allows adults the same type of comfort.

Journaling is the process of writing down thoughts as one experiences them. The journal is not meant for anyone else to read, and should contain thoughts on a particular subject along with initial reactions, the chosen behavior, and alternative options.

Deep breathing is highly recommended because it can be done anywhere at any time, often in conjunction with many of the other techniques. It is as simple as inhaling and exhaling.

Progressive relaxation entails the tightening and release of different parts of the body. There are several instructional tapes to guide the novice, or they can devise their own regimen.

Mental imagery is best described as a mental vacation. It involves closing one's eyes and picturing oneself somewhere, anywhere, more pleasant.

Finally, people can create their own methods. Most people have an idea of something that helps them relax or calm down. One caution to keep in mind: Some studies suggest that aggressive music stimulates an aggressive response to those listening, so it may be best to pick something soothing.

As adults, it is important for people to monitor the effects of stress, but it is equally important for parents to monitor the effects stress has on their children. Whether they are the one with aniridia or their child has aniridia, stress can and will impact their child if it is not dealt with appropriately. It is important for parents to remember that when they suffer from stress and exhibit a poor response, they model that same response to their child. It is very easy to displace frustration and anger onto our children, and when we do so, that is what we teach our children to do. Children learn from watching, and they watch their own parents most closely. The better parents become at identifying their stressors and applying appropriate remedies, the better it will be for their children, who will learn by example appropriate ways to resolve stress themselves.

It is important to recognize stress in children. Children will often display physical or behavioral changes when they are stressed. Physical effects typically include stomachaches, headaches, difficulty concentrating, and night terrors. Behavioral changes include mood swings, overreacting, acting out, attachment issues, bed-wetting, and changes in sleep or eating patterns. Younger children may also develop new habits such as thumb-sucking, hair-twirling or nose-picking; older children may begin to lie, bully, or defy authority figures.

Once it has been determined that a child is suffering from stress, the focus must shift to ways to help. Parents should prepare the child in advance for stressful situations such as doctor appointments or surgical procedures. The child will face the situation regardless, but if they are not given a change to express themselves, their level of anxiety will intensify with no chance of relief. As stated earlier, parents should model appropriate behavior. An effective way of doing this is by talking to their children about some of the parents' own concerns. It is okay to share with a child that they are scared or sad. Everyone gets scared and sad. There is no shame in admitting these natural feelings. Another helpful tool is to use appropriate books or programs to allow children to identify through characters. Parents can share a story with their child containing a theme that resembles his/her situation. Then they can allow the child to express how she or he feels about what happened. This is safe and nonthreatening for the child because the discussion is about the character and not the child. Finally, parents should establish and maintain daily "quality time." This provides the child with structure and an automatic stress-reliever. Although some children may appear to resist quality time, they also thrive on it, even though they may fail to recognize this on a conscious level.

In the end, it comes down to being proactive versus reactive. Is it better to prevent or respond? Choosing the latter means that not only does the stressor have to be dealt with, but so do the negative effects of stress. Choosing the former does not guarantee that all stress will be avoided, but it does lessen the chance of any negative effects.

There are several beneficial ways to be proactive. First, parents and patients should develop healthy habits and avoid irresponsible behavior. This means eating better, maintaining positive attitudes and feelings, talking to friends and family about issues or concerns as they arise, and avoiding depressing or over-stimulating news media and programs.

Second, parents and patients should develop realistic expectations and avoid perfectionism. The more realistic their expectations, the less likely they are to be disappointed. Also, perfection does not exist; therefore, there is no use in trying to obtain the impossible. Because people all have such busy lives, it is also helpful to prioritize and delegate tasks. In doing so, they should be flexible. Things may not get done their way, but they will get done. Along with this, it's a good idea for them to make to-do lists. They are a visual reminder that they are accomplishing their goals and making progress. Finally, they should be assertive. Sometimes one just has to say "no." It is much too draining to say "yes" all of the time. Until we find a way to clone ourselves, we must recognize our limitations for our sake and the sake of those around us.

Aniridia is a condition that will impact the lives of both those who have it and their family members. News of the condition is likely to bring about sadness, anger, confusion, and a variety of other feelings. The feelings are unavoidable and natural to the condition and the situations it creates. Having aniridia or a family member with aniridia is stressful; however, it does not have mean a life full of stress. There are ways to effectively deal with the stress and, at times, prevent stress from even occurring. Parents and patients need to identify the stressors in their life and how these impact them and those around them. Then they must ask themselves, "How do I want things to be different?" and, "In what ways can I make things different?" The only things that cannot be achieved are the things that the person does not try to achieve. Even if they try and are not successful, they should try again. There is more than one road leading to the final destination of a happy and stress-reduced life.

Notes

1. Clark, L. (1997). *SOS help for emotions: Managing anxiety, anger, and depression.* Bowling Green, KY: Parents Press.
2. Lebow, J. (2002). Transformation now! (or maybe later): Client change is not an all-or-nothing proposition. *Psychotherapy Networker,*. (Jan./Feb.), pp. 31–32.

9

Parents' Experiences

JESSICA J. OTIS

Children are the hands by which we take hold of heaven.

—Henry Ward Beecher

Editor's Note: Since not much was known about aniridia for many years some doctors did medical procedures that we now know should not be done on aniridic eyes. Please do not use any specific story here as a guide for your journey, because some of the medical procedures mentioned should not have been done. Furthermore, please make sure to see a doctor with experience and knowledge of anirida. Lastly, please keep in mind, each person's journey has different medical issues. Not everybody will experience the exact same medical challenges in their journeys.

When we face challenges in our lives, we turn to those who love and support us. Yet sometimes it isn't enough; we need the support of those who know how we are feeling and what we are going through. Parents who have children with aniridia can help each other by talking, lending advice, or just being there with a shoulder lean on. The stories compiled in this chapter are from parents who wish to share their personal experiences and struggles of having a child with aniridia. It is our wish that these stories will give you hope and inspiration as well as show you the love a parent has for a child, even when it seems like there is no light at the end of the tunnel.

KATHY, U.S.A. — LESSONS FROM THE HEART

When I was 29 years old, we were blessed with our third child. We already had two sons, and now we had a little girl! From the very beginning, I knew something was wrong. Amy seemed to keep her eyes closed most of the time. When I took her outdoors, she would bury her head in my shoulder. I told our pediatrician to look at her eyes, and he told us not to worry. He said that she had muscle problems that surgery could correct.

Over the months to follow, we decided to see an ophthalmologist. He told us that Amy had been born with a rare eye condition called aniridia. He said that her vision would be low and her eyes would be light-sensitive. Amy had muscle surgery to straighten the alignment of her eyes. She wore eye patches to strengthen her weak eye. Eyeglasses did not increase her vision, but dark glasses outdoors gave her relief from the bright light.

In elementary school, she was given large-print textbooks by the school system. Amy's vision up until this time had been 20/400 in one eye and 20/200 in her stronger eye. By the end of the seventh grade, both eyes were 20/400. It was very hard for Amy to keep up with the reading assigned because it strained her eyes. Many mornings she couldn't get them open enough to dress and go to school. We made the decision to home-school. Most of the teaching and learning was done orally. During this time, Amy was trained in computer skills and learned how to use visual aids. After graduating from high school, Amy had a great desire to go to college. After four years, she graduated with a degree in religious education. Today she is working as an administrative receptionist. Every day is a learning experience. Amy is a blessing to all who meet her.

I think the first time it really hit Amy that she was different was in her second year of elementary school. She had some glasses on her desk, and someone took them. When she entered the house, she began to sob. I prayed for wisdom. As I wiped her tears, I asked her if God ever made a mistake. She shook her head, "No." I continued, "And He didn't make a mistake when He created you either. You're no accident. He has a plan for your life." We've discovered through the years that everyone has "a disability"; while Amy's is visual, someone else's may be something that can't be seen, like anger, or fear, or jealousy, etc. We have had to learn how to deal with it and learn from it, and allow God to use it to make us the individuals He wants us to be.

One of the most radical decisions Amy made was to go away to college. We assumed she would attend the local university and live at home. When she announced that she had chosen an out-of-state college to attend, we were shocked. As we listened to her sharing her dream, we knew that we had to encourage her and help her be prepared for what was ahead. The August before she moved into the dorm, she attended a barbecue for the new students. She came home deva-stated. We both cried. It really hit her that night how hard it was going to be moving outside her comfort zone.

We wrote down all the things she was worried about. Would the teachers under-stand? Would she have any friends? Would she be able to find her classrooms? How would she get her food in the cafeteria? The list was a long one. When we finished, we read the list and asked God to meet her needs, and He did. But throughout the four years of college, there were many difficult days. I'll never forget one day Amy called and was sobbing. "It's too hard. I can't do it," she cried. Inside I was crying and my heart wanted to say I'd be there in an hour to bring her home, but I knew that wasn't the answer. I took a deep breath and listened as she shared her heartache. Then I prayed with her. She made it and grew stronger because of the tough times.

Any time we experience a loss or heartache, there are stages we go through emotionally: denial, anger, bargaining, depression, then acceptance. Each person works through these stages at his/her own pace. Moving through each stage brings healing. I believed at first that her vision could be fixed. I was angry with life and with God. I bargained and cried out, "Heal her, God." There were days of discouragement and fear. Acceptance is a hard thing, but it comes. I thank God for Amy, just the way she is! She is a fascinating young woman.

It's my faith in Jesus Christ that has carried me through each stage. The Bible and prayer have been my anchors. Without them, I couldn't cope. I would live in despair. There are still days of fear. The possibility that she will lose her vision altogether is always with us, but I know that God is always with us. He is faithful. When the doubts and fears flood my heart, I can give them to Him. Amy is learning the strength and courage that comes from fellowship with God. Praying for our children and praying with them are the greatest gifts we can give them. I can't always be with Amy, I can't solve all her problems, but I can point her to the one who can!

MARY, U.S.A. — HOW ANIRIDIA CAN AFFECT A FAMILY

Hello, my name is Mary. I would like to share with you my family and how aniridia has affected us. I live in a suburb just outside of Buffalo, New York, with my husband, Joe, and our five children, Joey, Alex, Marie, Madison, and Tori.

Tori is our youngest child at seventeen months old. At the age of six months she was diagnosed with sporadic aniridia. She was born full-term from a relatively uneventful pregnancy. Right before her six-month check up, we noticed we could see the red in her eyes when the light hit them just right. I also noticed that I could not define the color part (the iris) of her eye. I took her to the doctor, and the first thing she asked me was if I had any new questions or concerns. Of course, I said yes and proceeded to tell her my findings. She quickly took a look at Tori, and then made a call to the local pediatric ophthalmologist. After looking in her medical books and talking to him, she told me they believed Tori had aniridia. She told me a little bit about aniridia and WAGR syndrome, since Tori was a sporadic case. So we cut the regular visit short and got a sonogram to rule out the possibility of Wilms' tumor.

On a very personal note, I must say the next several weeks were quite an upsetting time. When I started to learn more and more about WAGR syndrome I became more anxious, nervous, and upset. You name the emotion, I had it. I read everything I could, and looked for every little thing that she did differently than my other children. After a long wait of two months to see the genetic doctors, we came to the conclusion that she only had sporadic aniridia. However, we still continue with the ultrasounds every three months. The urology team wants to stretch them to every four to six months, but I always tell them in a kind way that we will not extend the time between the ultrasounds. I continue to tell them she will have the ultrasounds every three months until she is about six or seven years old. After that she will continue with them every six months for several years.

In addition, I would like to share my emotional experience of having a child diagnosed with sporadic aniridia. I believe that when something like aniridia is passed on, it is much different for that family, and parents in particular, than it is for someone who has a new case of it. I cannot share with you how it affects inherited cases, but I can tell you for me and my family how it has affected us. When she was first diagnosed, and before I knew very much about aniridia, I went into a state of depression and unimaginable pain. Not pain for myself so much, but for my daughter. I think I cried for about two weeks straight. I looked for reasons everywhere and anywhere. I asked, "Why?" I just wanted to know why. So I looked for the answers and did not find many. Over time I have come to the conclusion that I love my daughter just the way she is and I would not change her in any way. Okay, I might ask for some brand new irises and such, but you know what I mean. I have learned to take it one day, one week, one month, and one year at a time. Every six months she visits the ophthalmologist, and I say to myself *six months down and no new problems*. I'll take every six months that I can get, and be very grateful for each of them. There are several worse things out there, so I am glad my daughter only has aniridia. And for that I thank God.

Today Tori is a happy and healthy seventeen-month-old little girl. She is walking and talking more and more each day. She gets into her fair share of trouble around the house. Keeping up with four older brothers and sisters is a big job. Tori amazes me every day, and she does a lot more than I thought she would be able to do for her age, given the visual impairment. We do not know what her visual acuity is yet, but so far she has no cataracts, signs of glaucoma, or corneal pannus.

To the families of new children born with aniridia, I just want to say that it does get easier over time. That does not mean it goes away. I still think about her and her eyes almost every minute, but it is part of her life—and ours, for that matter. I will be the best advocate for her that I can be, and I will teach her to be the same for herself.

Lastly, I would like to say Aniridia Foundation International has been such a great support system for our family and is also very informative. If all members could work together, just imagine what we could accomplish.

T.L., U.S.A.—DIFFICULTIES RAISING A CHILD WITH ANIRIDIA

I was born and raised in Milwaukee, Wisconsin, and live in Brown Deer, a suburb of Milwaukee. I have a 20-year-old daughter with sporadic aniridia. She was also born with cataracts in both eyes, and developed glaucoma at age eight. She has had numerous surgeries, starting at age nine months for the removal of her cataracts, and as recently as six weeks ago for a detached retina. She had a Barveldt valve put in a year ago for glaucoma. She would like to have a stem cell and corneal transplant, but is very nervous about it. She just gave birth in October to a son, who fortunately doesn't have aniridia. My daughter wasn't diagnosed until she was three months old, and then it was by a pediatrician, not the ophthalmologist I had taken her to see. I was lucky that we have an eye institute to take her to, but they were pretty much guessing about how to treat her. I had my son one week after a redo of the cataract surgery, and brought him with us for our first post-op appointment. He didn't have aniridia. It was a struggle with every-thing regarding my daughter, because we didn't know what to expect, and we had no one else to talk to with the same experience. My daughter went to a Catholic grade school, and two years of Catholic high school. She always had low grades because the teachers provided no extra time or any help. She rebelled at sixteen years old, and it wasn't until then that we discovered she could have an IEP [Individualized Education Program]. We sent her to a small private high school, where with the proper help and visual aids she was able to graduate at age seventeen. My daughter was able to get a restricted driver's license, and drove for about three years until she developed corneal scarring. She was able to get a degree in early childhood development, and worked at a daycare for several years. Today she is married and lives in Richland Center, Wisconsin.

My husband and I have gone to every Aniridia Foundation International conference, and it has made a big difference in our lives. When I first saw others with aniridia, I wanted to cry, because I finally knew my daughter wasn't the only one with it. I have learned so much information that I never knew before. In talking with one of the moms whose daughter is about the same age as mine, I told her I had thought that I was the cause of my daughter's aniridia. I had gone into a hot tub while I was pregnant, and I actually thought I'd burned her irises off! I felt guilty all of those years. That mom said she had thought the same thing. It was just such a relief to hear that someone shared my feelings. We are so glad that a foundation was started. My advice for new parents would be to join this group and attend the conferences.

JAMIE, U.S.A.—HOPE AND ENCOURAGEMENT
(CHILD WITH WAGR SYNDROME)

I'll never forget the fear I had inside me hearing what it all meant when our son, Dylan, was diagnosed with aniridia and WAGR syndrome. I remember thinking about all the things he'll never be able to do or enjoy, like play baseball or even see a star. The first six months of his life, he showed very little interest in objects or even us. At that time, I decided to enroll in a Hadley School for the Blind online class for parents who had a visually impaired child. That course empowered me to see the possibilities and opportunities my son will have, and it also included a great resource guide that can be used throughout his life. Soon after, Dylan started to show interest in objects and us! It was like someone turning on the light for him.

He is currently six years old and has taught us more than I could ever imagine. He has battled Wilms' tumor twice, and had multiple surgeries over the past years. Nothing stops him. He's the happiest kid I know. We're there to guide him and encourage him to do the things he wants to do and always help him along the way. With a little modification, there is nothing he won't be able to do, even see a star.

JANELL, U.S.A.—NEVER LOSE HOPE!

I have a seven-year-old son named Kyle. He was diagnosed with sporadic aniridia when he was two months old. Along with aniridia he also has nystagmus, glaucoma, microscopic cataracts, and degenerative maculas. When Kyle was first diagnosed with aniridia, we were devastated. We couldn't even remember what it was called for the first few days. We eventually learned more about it, and even found out about two people that have aniridia, and got to talk to them. Also, we have had a very supportive family, friends, and church. I personally find comfort from reading my Bible and attending the ladies' Bible study groups at our church. I know that God has a special plan and purpose for everyone, even people with disabilities. Sometimes we find out what that purpose is right away, and sometimes we don't. My husband and I have become better people, and more compassionate and concerned for people with different "challenges" than others, since we had Kyle. I have a very soft spot in my heart for these people, especially the children. I am always curious to talk with parents of children with disabilities, because I've been there and I know how difficult it can be. Another thing that has happened as a result of Kyle's aniridia and other vision problems is that I have been able to help and comfort other people whose children have vision problems or other disabilities. As I said before, God has a special plan and purpose for everyone He creates. It's our responsibility to work through our challenges every day to the best of our ability, knowing He is still in control.

In the beginning it was hard at times when we'd drop Kyle off at the church nursery when he was younger. One time they had a fire drill and the teachers got in a hurry with the kids and took Kyle out without his sunglasses. My sister-in-law worked in the children's ministry at the time, and she saw him with his class and without his sunglasses. So she rushed back in to get his glasses from the classroom. It was hard putting him in PPCD (Preschool Program for Children with Disabilities) and kindergarten too, because we had to explain the seriousness of his wearing his sunglasses outside, even if it's raining outside. It was always hard to leave him someplace new because we were afraid the people working with him would forget about things that would seem minor to anyone else.

Today Kyle has about 20/200 visual acuity and wears glasses at school and when he does schoolwork. However, his eyes tire easily because of the nystagmus, so he takes a lot of breaks when he's doing homework, and the school has shortened his handwriting assignments. They also give him breaks during the day, and he has an aide in the classroom to assist him when needed. He does very well with reading and math. He was in a PPCD class for three years and had a wonderful teacher, but now he's only in first grade, so I don't have very much information on school progress yet. Kyle has acted pretty much like other kids, but he was a little slower at some things. He has fine-motor difficulties, some gross-motor delays, and some tactile defensiveness. Kyle also has AD/HD (attention-deficit/hyperactivity disorder) and possibly a slight form of PDD/NOS (pervasive developmental disorder—not otherwise specified).

Finally, I'd just like to tell all the parents out there to never lose hope! Take every day and every challenge one at a time. Remember God is in control, and He has a unique plan and purpose for that special person in your life. You just have to wait and see what He will do with and through that person. Having a child with special "challenges" isn't what we expect or hope for, but we can learn from it and benefit from it. God doesn't give these special children to just anyone. He hand-selects the special parents for these children. We should feel honored that God saw something special and different enough in us to give us this opportunity. If you have a child with aniridia, don't ask "Why?" even if you don't understand it. Being a parent of a child with special needs isn't easy: it is a challenge, but it's also a blessing. A very delicate blessing that oftentimes goes unnoticed by the general public. Despite the difficulties we experience having a child or children with special needs, I feel that in the long run we will see that it was well worth it. We will have accomplished a very rewarding task that goes far beyond the basic principles of parenthood. We will learn to thank God for giving us the special responsibility of loving and bringing up this special little person. We are the honored parents. Praise God for His special plan for all of us!

DAWN, U.S.A.—EXPLAINING ANIRIDIA TO OTHERS

Our daughter was diagnosed at five months old with what doctors thought to be sporadic aniridia. From the age of two months she showed evidence of vertical nystagmus, but the doctor said it would get better as she got older. We only see it a little now when she is extremely fatigued. When she was first diagnosed, we were scared, not sure what "aniridia" meant, and a bit frightened by how important it is to protect her vision. We felt as though it was somehow our fault. Even though it was not something that ran in our family, we felt we had done this to her. We asked ourselves, how were we going to deal with what her future would be like?

Her vision is now improving each time we go to the ophthalmologist, and although we know it won't be 20/20 without glasses, we know she can see a lot more than we expected her to be able to see. She accomplishes new developmental milestones each and every day. We know it is something we had no control over. We know we'll always be here for her no matter what hurdles she'll have to cross in the future. She is such a beautiful little girl, and we would not trade her for the world!

One struggle we have gone through is explaining her condition to others. At first, we'd get upset when people commented on how "sleepy" she looked. That is a byproduct of how an aniridic blocks out unwanted light. Now, we sometimes just agree with them and say, "Yes, it's almost naptime." People just don't understand her eye condition and often pity her when we do explain it. Pity is not what we want for her. We want her to be accepted for herself and all her accomplishments and not her condition.

Currently, she has been diagnosed with Gillespie's syndrome, which involves the eyes and brain (a part of the brain that controls balance and coordination). She also is unable to walk without the assistance of equipment due to the cerebellar ataxia, but she gets stronger each and every day.

The best advice I can give other parents is to rely on a support system (husband, wife, friends, and relatives). Get help with caring for your child so you, as a parent, can have a little time to yourself. It's important to take a breather now and then because you can get burned out pretty quickly, and you're not much good if you don't take the time to recharge. Also try to take the days one at a time and cherish your child with aniridia, because he or she is a precious gift.

S.P., LIECHTENSTEIN—DON'T WORRY!

We live in Liechtenstein and have a three-year-old daughter. At seven weeks old my daughter was diagnosed with sporadic aniridia. I was shocked and over-whelmed, and at the same time I felt that I needed to be strong for her. I did not know what this diagnosis meant exactly. I didn't know if I was able to give her the right kind of care. I was scared that she would not be accepted by society with this eye condition. I felt lost and lonely because I didn't know anyone with the same condition. Then I found the Aniridia Foundation International and International Aniridia Network websites. All the postings on these networks have helped me a great deal in learning how to give my daughter the best care possible. I find the networks very inspiring and important for everyone. From being able to read information and postings on these sites I learned more about aniridia, and now I understand it enough to explain it to others. Also, I'm fine with her condition. She has therapy twice a week, and I work with her a lot at home ("homework" from therapy). She goes to several checkups every three months, and her development gives me great encouragement. She is developing beautifully, and I'm convinced that she will find her way in this world. To other parents out there, please do not let this condition rule your life, make it part of your family life! *Do not worry!* Raise your child the same way you would raise any child, and keep in mind that every day your child accomplishes a great deal with little vision. Once in a while, close your eyes and try to imagine how this (new) situation would affect you, if you couldn't see well. Be patient with your child, and you will see wonderful things happening.

KIRSTEN, DENMARK—AWARENESS

My daughter Nina was born with sporadic aniridia in 1992. When we went to see a pediatrician for her allergy, I asked her to take an extra look at Nina's eyes. She was then almost a year old. I had tried to reason with our local doctor and told him that there was something funny about her eye color, which turned red like the eyes of a dog when light came into them. He asked if there had been ancestors with darker eyes (which there had) and just told me that since her hair was red (different from the rest of our family), her eyes were just very dark brown and not to worry. When she was finally diagnosed with aniridia, I was devastated for some time. I cried and cried. Our first child had been stillborn. Then we had a completely healthy girl, who was almost three years old, and now this "handi-capped" child. I felt cursed in some way, and then I went into "action mode" and started to investigate and research the condition (I'm a journalist by profession).

It was pretty difficult to get knowledge at that time, because Denmark has a population of just five million and there was only one medical study of the condition. It was written during the 1930s and sort of concluded that there was nothing to do about it, and that the condition was often accompanied by low intelligence. The doctor who lent it to me told me this and said that he was of a different opinion, but I insisted on reading it. I then phoned the medical research center of the Panum Institute (University of Copenhagen) and asked them to make a search of the Internet, which was not at that time the everyday item that it is today. They supplied me with data and references, which I then searched for more details. That was how I first heard of the risk for Wilms' tumor and was able to tell the eye specialist about this risk. That was news for him! We then got frequent screenings for a year or two. Nothing was ever found. Now apart from buying the medicine (drops) to treat Nina's eyes and reminding her to wear glasses/sunglasses, I don't think very much about it. It's part of our lives. But now that she is getting older, I have started to think about her choices of education and her future possibilities when it comes to employment.

Today in school she is doing quite well without any real need for help. At least she didn't want any until recently, when she got a special computer that can enlarge text and has a reading program so she can listen to text instead of getting tired from glancing at the screen. I've tried to help her get novels and larger pieces of reading on tapes, but she wants to be treated like anybody else. Which gives us some discussions. She has a lot of friends and social activities, and rides her bike to school every day. This school year she spends her days with 109 other Danish students at a school that is 110 kilometers from our home. So she's had to get acquainted with them and fall into the group, and it seems to work just fine. At her new school they use whiteboards and projectors instead of old-fashioned chalkboards, and she likes that much better. She is still placed in the front of the classroom, but now knows that it is in her best interest. My number-one piece of advice to parents is to be aware of the condition, to try to help as best you can, but don't make it more of a problem than it is.

CHRISTY, U.S.A.—CHILD HAVING SURGERIES

My daughter Carrie is seven years old and was born with sporadic aniridia. Carrie also has nystagmus, cataracts, and glaucoma. When she was born, we noticed her eyes looked different (a very strange ice-cold blue color). Later we were told it was caused by glaucoma that gave her high eye pressures at birth, but we didn't really know why or that it was something serious. We went to a new pediatrician forty-eight hours after her birth, and he sent us to a pediatric ophthalmologist. Then he sent us to a corneal specialist at LeBonhuer Children's Hospital who gave us the final news. All the other doctors said they thought it was something called aniridia, but they weren't sure because they had never actually seen it before. One doctor said he had been practicing over thirty years and had never seen it until that day. So Carrie was two days old when we really knew for sure what she had and what it was called. When we heard about the condition, we were devastated. All we knew were the horrible things that could accompany this eye condition, since it affects far more than just the eyes. So many children have so much more. Some children even can die from the related conditions. Over time we have learned that this disease is not what you would ever wish for anyone to live with, especially not your child. But people must get on with their lives and learn to adapt, learn new skills, dream up a new life with a new future, and realize that no matter how hard you have it, there is always someone who has it worse than you do. It may seem hard to do, but after so many trips to the special care unit for little babies six months and under, after her surgeries I saw some children in there when I was feeling pretty down about my own, and I realized many times over to be thankful that my child was not as bad off as many of them were.

This brings me to all the surgeries Carrie has undergone. Starting at the age of two weeks old she had her first surgery for the glaucoma in her left eye. Then at four weeks old she had the same surgery on her right eye. She has had lots of scar tissue removed at EUAs (examination under anesthesia), and eventually she had tubes put in both eyes for the glaucoma. Then she had a corneal transplant, and it failed about two months later. After that the doctors found that a corneal transplant without a stem cell transplant as well would always fail. So we tried again, having the corneal transplant with the stem cells as well, but it failed quicker than the first time. This time it only lasted about a month. It was very discouraging. After the second surgery we were told that with every rejection the chances decrease of another one working. I believe we are through with surgeries for now.

Today Carrie works extra hard at home and she stays on task and grade level. She used to spend part of her day in resource and part of the day in the regular classroom, but now she is in her regular class full-time. Carrie has accomplished so much! She can do anything she sets her mind to do. She is learning to play the piano and is doing great. She is one of the top three children in her regular classroom. She loves to sing and is great at it. I believe this child will do great things in her life and show others that even with a huge handicap it can be done. So the one thing I would like parents to remember is to just learn all you can. Talk with other families, get advice, and do what you think is best for your child. And above all else, love your child!

STACY, U.S.A.—ALL I EVER NEEDED

Just shy of three years ago, I knew what I wanted from life. Life was even sweeter with the anticipation of the arrival of our first child. Even though life was as close to where I wanted it to be as ever, I still did not know what I needed . . . . until Adison.

My husband, Adam, has aniridia (the first in his family). It always seemed a secondary issue, almost a non-issue. I had almost forgotten about this until soon after Adison was born, when our pediatrician expressed her concern over our beautiful girl's "huge red light reflex." It hit me all at once: no iris, our six-pound dream with dimples and mop of dark hair also has her daddy's eyes, and aniridia.

I trudged through life with the diagnosis hanging over us, just waiting for everything to cave in. Day by day, things seemed—dare I say?—normal. We knew Adison cried a lot, slept little, had pronounced nystagmus, and needed near-constant physical contact, but she seemed to be meeting her developmental milestones. It was not until her first EUA at seven months old that our "normalcy" was disrupted.

Our then-ophthalmologist informed us her pressures were normal, and he had performed a prophylactic goniotomy on both eyes, but he was "impressed" by the corneal pannus already present. He flatly stated we could expect her to lose her vision by early adulthood. I could not move out of that cold hard chair in the waiting room. I decided right then and there, I would do whatever I needed to rally help for my daughter. I had never even heard of corneal pannus before that moment.

It took numerous phone calls and being mildly "pushy" to enlist help, but it was well worth the tears and frustration. We became involved with Early Intervention and with the Toddler Program at the Western Pennsylvania School for Blind Children. Now, as I look at my almost three-year-old dream, I see her, not aniridia. I see a beautiful, smart, funny, brave, and fiercely independent little girl with a smile and imagination that light up my world. She is in a three-year-old preschool class, loves her ballet class and Dora the Explorer, and is easily frustrated by her eighteen-month-old brother Nathan (without aniridia). She is the joy of my heart and life. She is the reason I am here. As we get ready to celebrate her third birthday, we are celebrating another year of hope, triumph, and looking toward a bright future. All I ever needed was Adison, to show me what it is to be a mom and how to love with my whole being, and that what you want is always less important than what you need.

MARK AND JENNIFER, U.S.A. — SHE'S PERFECT (CHILD WITH WAGR SYNDROME)

During my wife's pregnancy, she and I journeyed on a roller coaster of emotions. Early on in the pregnancy we were told there was a chance our baby could be born with some kind of chromosomal abnormality. For peace of mind, we had additional tests performed to rule out any abnormalities, and fortunately they did. We felt as though we had bypassed any bad news. Then on April 15, 2004, Jennifer gave birth to our little angel, Kadina Marie, and the emotional ride finally had ended on a good note . . . or so we thought.

Looking at Kadina, she appeared to be the most flawless baby I had ever seen. She was 18 inches and six pounds, five ounces of pure perfection. Her skin glowed as if every angel in heaven blanketed her in kisses. She was truly a sight, and I knew that the beauty we saw before us was only the beginning. Her inner beauty had yet to be seen, but when given the opportunity, it would shine as though she were lighting up the world.

That first day, all I cared about was getting to know my daughter. I remember thinking many things. "What kind of person will she become?" "What sports will she play?" "Who will be her favorite cartoon character?" True, I had no idea what the answers would be, but the questions (even though they were premature) were fun to think about. Then during Kadina's second day in this world, my wife and I were given an answer as to what kind of person our daughter would be: a fighter.

On April 16, the day after my greatest day ever, a doctor came to examine my little girl. My wife and I remained optimistic and believed that everything would be fine, but from the doctor's news, things were not fine. He told us that Kadina had a rare eye condition: aniridia, as we've come to know it. We were also informed she would need further testing because she could be at risk for another condition, WAGR syndrome. Upon further testing it was discovered that Kadina does have WAGR syndrome, and the news went from bad to worse.

At this point the roller coaster ride had become exhausting, but little did we know that the greatest plunge had yet to come. On September 7, 2007, Kadina was diagnosed with a Wilms' tumor on her right kidney. Despite all the talks with doctors and knowledge we had been given, nothing could prepare us for this news. This was news I didn't think I could survive, but I knew I couldn't give up because my little inspiration hadn't given up. I just had to find the strength and courage she already possessed.

The transformation happened so quickly. Within no time at all the thick curls that had once covered her precious little head had fallen out, leaving nothing but smooth skin. Soon she began to lose weight and withered to next to nothing, but still Kadina never lost her smile. Week after week we had to endure a two-hour car ride to go for treatments certain to make her feel sick, but still, she never lost her smile. Nothing could break this little girl's spirit because she is a fighter, and no fighter ever takes on a battle believing they are going to lose. Kadina is no exception. Time and time again she has prevailed over all of life's challenges in victorious fashion, and she always did it with a smile on her face.

The diagnosis was most difficult to accept, and filled Jennifer and me with much anger and sadness. Nevertheless, miraculously the clouds that had over-taken our lives parted, and the sun began to shine, all from one simple gesture, a smile. My daughter's smile represents her strength and ability to fight. When she smiles, it's her way of saying, "Daddy, don't be sad, because I'm happy." Because of that I have been able to let go of the anger and sadness. All I have ever wanted is a happy and healthy child. Happy she is without a doubt. As for healthy, that can be debated by some. True, her eyes are not perfect, but neither are my eyes. True, she had a cancerous mass removed from her, but her body continues to heal and get stronger. I have learned that although my daughter is different, she is more the same. I accept the gift God has given me and wouldn't exchange her for the world. Even though her eyes are the darkest of colors, when I look into them they light up my life. Kadina is no less perfect than that first moment I saw her.

VICTORIA AND CRAIG, NEW ZEALAND—HAVING YOUR CHILD DIAGNOSED WITH ANIRIDIA

May 10, 2004 was an amazing day! I gave birth to our first baby. We had a beautiful dark-haired son whom we named William (Will). He was born three weeks early, so he was on the small side at five pounds, seven ounces, but he was pronounced healthy and well, with everything intact and as it should be. We took him home and began our new family life, blissfully unaware of what was in store for us in the weeks to come.

Life with Will at home was great. He was a good baby who ate, slept, and did everything as he should. My midwife visited him every week for the first six weeks, and she pronounced him a thriving baby boy. She didn't notice anything unusual with his eyes, as he actually had them closed for the majority of the time.

When he did briefly open them, Craig and I couldn't tell what color his eyes were, but naïvely thought that all babies started off with dark eyes and the color would come later. Our postnatal care was handed over to the district nurse after six weeks (common practice in New Zealand), and it was on her second visit that she noticed Will occasionally rolled his eyes and did not focus or track objects as he should. We were told to take Will to our local doctor, so we did that very afternoon.

The doctor was not overly familiar with eye conditions, but she did think she saw a small cataract in Will's right eye. She referred us to a pediatric ophthalmologist, but the appointment was not for two weeks. Now we were getting quite worried and starting to think something could be seriously wrong. My husband Craig was more optimistic, thinking it was something that could be fixed by glasses or surgery, but we were both nervous enough to not be able to wait two whole weeks to find out for sure. Faxes and phone calls were made to the specialist's office expressing our deep worry and requesting an earlier appointment. The appointment was changed, and we saw the ophthalmologist four days later on July 16, 2004. Will was nine weeks old.

I can confidently say that July 16, 2004, was the worst day of our lives so far. It still brings me to tears just thinking about that day. It was the day we found out that our perfect, darling, nine-week-old son, Will, was not what we thought. The ophthalmologist looked at some video we had taken of Will at home, as oddly enough, his eyes didn't bounce at all in the doctor's office. She then laid Will on the floor and examined his eyes. As she got up, she said, "I don't think Will has any irises in his eyes." What that meant was beyond us. In silence we picked up Will from the floor, and my mother held him as we heard the doctor tell us, "William has an extremely rare genetic condition called aniridia. Aniridia literally means 'without an iris.' That in itself is not the main problem. The back of his eye has not developed properly, and it is very likely he will have extremely poor vision. You must also get him screened for a kidney cancer called Wilms' tumor, and a brain scan is also necessary since Wilms' tumor, mental retardation, and genital anomalies are all conditions linked with aniridia." By this stage I was in complete shock and didn't speak at all. Craig asked a few questions, and we left the doctor's office that Friday afternoon feeling numb with disbelief at what we had just heard. We were left carrying a baby to the car who was now not our darling, sweet, perfect baby, but possibly a blind mentally retarded baby who might also have cancer. Life couldn't have gotten any worse.

We drove home in virtual silence, each of us not knowing what to say. I felt overcome with grief, but I couldn't cry. It was not until two days later that I managed some tears and felt the full impact of what we had been told. It felt as though my world as I knew it had fallen apart, and I had come up against something that I didn't know how to recover from. I had no idea how I would care for this damaged baby, and to be honest I didn't even want to care for him anymore. I could no longer breastfeed him, so he was weaned to the bottle. I didn't get up for him when he cried in the night; my mother and sister took over this role as they came and stayed for a week after the diagnosis. The grief was overwhelming, I really felt like I couldn't continue living, and seeing my eternally positive and strong husband crumble into tears was just so painful. I think my main sadness came from the fact that I felt I had failed, failed to produce a perfect healthy baby like everyone else does. We asked, "Why us?" over and over, and there was just no answer. Our local doctor came over and offered support and the reassurance that she didn't think Will had any mental problems as his muscle tone was so good. He also moved his hands to the midline, which was also a big developmental step.

We researched aniridia on the Internet (after learning how to spell it!), which I must say did more damage than it needed to do. We didn't know what we were reading and if it applied to Will specifically. WAGR syndrome was mentioned, and that was obviously what the doctors would be looking for at his upcoming appointment. We spoke to the lady who was to become Will's vision teacher from the regional School for the Blind and Visually Impaired, and also to an acquaintance who has a son with a genetic eye problem. Speaking to her was amazing. She gave us hope and made us see that Will was still the perfect, wee baby we had had all along. It's just that now he may face other challenges in his life. So after gathering information, talking to people, and preparing ourselves for the worst, we sat tight through a tense, heart-wrenching, and tearful few days while we awaited the hospital visit.

The next Wednesday we went to Starship Children's Hospital in Auckland for an MRI scan of Will's brain, an ultrasound of his kidneys, and to have some blood taken. Thankfully all went well, and he was given a perfect bill of health from both the MRI and ultrasound. That was a huge relief! The ultrasounds would continue every three months, but for now he was fine and didn't have cancer. That was cause for celebration when we got home! Next came a meeting with a geneticist who explained all the genetic implications of aniridia for Will's having children, for our having more children, and the testing that could be done to find out exactly what mutation had occurred in Will's genetic makeup. Craig and I had a thorough eye examination in which they were looking for any subtle signs of aniridia that may have manifested itself in our eyes, but not have any effect on our eyesight. The tests were all clear and our eyes were fine.

Some of Will's blood was sent to a lab in Texas, United States, for DNA testing to see if they could identify whether his kidney gene had also been affected and therefore predict the likelihood of his contracting Wilms' tumor later on. Although they gave no guarantee that he absolutely could not get Wilms', they did say he was extremely unlikely to get it since his kidney gene was unaffected. Ultrasound screening was no longer medically necessary, according to the doctors, but Craig and I have opted to continue screening Will every six months; after all he is our baby, not theirs, and there is no 100 percent guarantee offered that he won't get Wilms'. Now at least we knew for sure that Will only had isolated aniridia (not WAGR syndrome).

More blood was sent to a lab in Edinburgh, Scotland, to be tested to see if they could locate the exact mutation that had occurred in Will's genes and caused the aniridia. This was also successful and the exact mutation was discovered. It was a mutation they had not encountered before, unique to Will, so they asked that Craig and I send some bloods for testing also. We are awaiting these results, but it may be able to tell us if we are mosaic carriers; that is, whether some of either our eggs or sperm are carrying the aniridia gene. It could be any number of my eggs or Craig's sperm that carry it, or it could be none at all. In any case, for future pregnancies we have been offered the chance to have a CVS (chorionic villus sampling) test done at twelve weeks, which would show for sure whether that baby also had aniridia.

The aniridia network websites in the United States and the United Kingdom have been extremely helpful, especially with the support offered from other mothers whose children are a bit older and therefore a few steps ahead of where we are right now. It is great to know what to expect in the future. Just yesterday I got an email from a distraught grandmother whose three-month-old grand-daughter had just been diagnosed with aniridia. She got my name from an aniridia website, so that shows the good that comes of forming support networks, especially for a condition that doesn't occur very often.

Will continues to grow and thrive. He crawled at nine months, and he is eating finger food and picking up small objects such as peas and raisins from his high-chair tray. He loves to clap hands, pull himself to a stand, and have cuddles. He crawls all over the house exploring everywhere. He is not particular about what he touches. He loves playing in sand, crawls on the grass, and mashes up jelly and fruit with no problems. He has swimming lessons, which he adores, almost as much as playing in the bottom of the shower! In all, he is developing wonderfully and we have no concerns that he will have anything other than a happy and fulfilling life. He is a very loved little boy by the whole extended family and we wouldn't have him any other way.

CARRIE, U.S.A.—LITTLE BLACK-EYED PEA

The day I was born, 28 years ago, my parents were told that I was blind. Months later, my mom figured out that I had vision when I started to grab objects. Reflecting back on my childhood, I do remember being different from the other children. In first grade I was running on the playground and smacked into the monkey bars. I told my mom that because I had to shut my eyes, I could not see the playground equipment until it was too late. I had a vision teacher, large-print books, and special equipment. The older I became the more I hated the attention that came along with low vision. In fact, it was never the low vision itself or the light sensitivity that bothered me, it was people treating me like I was helpless. I learned how to compensate for what I could not see, and actually told everyone I could see fine. I choose to play soccer instead of softball and just learned the ball was probably where everyone was running to. I just "forgot" that I had aniridia and lived my life. I graduated from college, got married, and had a son.

Then my daughter was born. A few hours after she was born, the doctor was examining her. He looked into her eyes and I knew by his look something was wrong. He told me he thought she had a drug overdose, and I explained to him that it was "just" aniridia. I quickly educated him on aniridia in the very casual conversation, and he left the hospital room to go do research. I sat there all alone with my daughter and looked at her. I cannot put into words the emotional overload I felt. I was scared, sad, and grateful all at the same time. I felt guilty because I had a perfectly healthy girl with all her major organs working and some other parents would do anything to be in this situation. I felt heartbroken because I know firsthand the challenges my daughter will face throughout her life. I just sat there with my daughter and cried. This might sound crazy to people, but I felt at peace holding her. I know that as long as I have her in my life, everything will be fine.

My parents' approach to coping with this was amazing considering there was little knowledge about aniridia at that time. The best gift my parents gave me was expecting me to be independent, not just saying it but truly believing it was possible. I know now that I am a role model, and my attitude and outlook towards this is crucial for my daughter's emotional well-being. For example, she has a predominant nystagmus. There have been several rude comments to us in public. Initially, I have a maternal instinct like a mother bear protecting her cub; however, I know my reaction to these situations teaches her to be confident, direct, and respectful to others. I hope that this approach will bring harmony to her life as opposed to fighting her way through this sometimes critical and harsh world.

My perception of the seriousness of aniridia has changed since the arrival of my daughter. My curiosity for knowledge is endless, and I am hopeful for our future. I love my little black-eyed pea.

SHIPRA, INDIA—DIFFERENT SOCIETY VIEW

August 18, 2005, was the day I encountered the biggest trial of my life. My younger daughter was born that day, and when she was only five hours old the doctor informed us that she had aniridia. My husband and I thought, "ani—ridia?" That was the first time we heard this term *aniridia*. We knew nothing about it, and we were also informed she might be legally blind, The work "blind" hit us so badly that even all the medication the nurse provided could not help me sleep.

We are from India. We were planning on moving back to India after the birth of our daughter. But after we received this news we began to think, should we take our daughter to India? India is a developing nation, and has its own social evils. One of them is the treatment of the handicapped! People and even their families are looked down on if they have a handicap. I can remember when I was growing up there was a blind lady living in our neighborhood. I always saw her struggling all her life. Her family did not support her, no one married her, and some kids in the neighborhood used to tease her and sometimes threw stones at her! This made us wonder, will our daughter and our family be treated like this in these circumstances?

The bottom line is that Indian society might not accept this, so we decided to stay here. Now our baby is three and a half years old. People here treat her the same way they would treat any three-year-old. We are very lucky that we live in America.

CYNTHIA, U.S.A.—THREE GENERATIONS

On November 1, 1957, a healthy baby girl, Cynthia, was placed in the arms of parents, Dorothy and Francis. It was not until Cynthia was almost one year old that her maternal aunt, Myrtle, noticed something different about her eyes. With great concern, Dorothy took her baby girl to a local ophthalmologist. He told Cynthia's parents that she had a *coloboma* (a catch-all term meaning "a hole in an eye structure") but her eyes were okay. Cynthia's eye had a small absence of her iris. Cynthia's parents continued to watch her eyesight. Cynthia has progressed through most of her life with 20/20 vision. It wasn't until 1997 that Cynthia began to wear bifocals. She was working as an auditor for the state and teaching college four nights a week. On June 8, 2003, Dr. Edward Holland confirmed that Cynthia (age 45) did indeed have a mild case of aniridia. In July 2004, another ophthalmologist told Cynthia that she has borderline glaucoma.

On September 29, 1977, two years after Cynthia married Dennis, she had a beautiful baby girl, Michelle. Her pediatrician noticed her irises and asked her ophthalmologist to examine Michelle. He talked with Cynthia privately, and told her that the prognosis for Michelle's eyesight was poor. He said that if Cynthia and Dennis had any more children, there would be a 50/50 chance they too would have aniridia. He recommended that we reconsider having more children. He asked to examine her at one month, four months, one year, and every year thereafter. As Michelle grew, eye examinations showed that she had nystagmus, 20/200 visual acuity, and a small stub of an iris. He said she basically had no iris.

Cynthia was asked to bring Michelle to the Southern College of Optometry in Memphis, Tennessee, when she was three years old. At this visit, an EEG was performed that showed that Michelle had better vision in her left eye, but the nystagmus was worse. In the right eye, the nystagmus was better, but the vision was worse.

Her eyesight remained basically the same until she was hit in the right eye with a volleyball in the eight grade (1991). Seven months later, Michelle was diagnosed with glaucoma. She immediately started a regimen of Timoptic. Michelle's glaucoma diagnosis was difficult for Cynthia. Her coping mechanism was to research aniridia more thoroughly. It was during these studies that she learned of WAGR syndrome and its ramifications. Cynthia found out Michelle was at risk for Wilms' tumor, and that the risk was higher for her up to three years of age. From then on, Cynthia made sure Michelle had annual ultrasounds.

In 1993, at the age of sixteen, Michelle visited the Southern College of Optometry and was told that she could meet the criteria to be a licensed driver using bioptic glasses. Michelle had to go to a local optometrist for eight visits to learn how to use the bioptic glasses to drive. Then she took driver's education courses and training to drive. After completion of the training and courses, her physician gave her his authorization for the eye test portion of the test. With approval in hand, Michelle took and passed the written and driving portion of the test. Michelle received a Class D license. Her license has to be recertified annually after her annual eye exam.

In the spring of 1994, the eye pressure in her right eye started to fluctuate. Dr. Lowe increased her medication. In August 1994, after a prescription regimen of eight different medications, with increased eye pressure, she was referred to Vanderbilt University Medical Center. In October 1994, Michelle had a trabulectomy on her right eye. Immediately after the surgery, the doctor told Cynthia that the surgery would probably not work, but that it was the first step. Six weeks later Cynthia was told that it had worked. She was so thrilled she asked if she could make presentations at medical conferences about her success.

Michelle was mainstreamed into regular public classrooms until the spring of her junior year. After her surgery, Michelle's itinerant teacher felt it would be good for her to transfer to the Tennessee School for the Blind. Michelle graduated second in her class at the Tennessee School for the Blind.

Michelle's eyesight and pressure stabilized until May 2001, when she developed eye ulcers. In February 2003, Dr. Edward Holland first examined Michelle. Dr. Holland told her that she needed the KLAL [keratolimbal allograft] stem cell surgery. In preparation for this surgery, he suggested that she have her local ophthalmologist place a shunt in her eye. The shunt surgery went well. After recuperating, as a military dependent, Michelle had to consult her local military ophthalmologist. Her insurance would not cover her surgery. One year later and after Michelle's divorce, Medicaid approved the procedure. With Medicaid coverage, Michelle received approval for Dr. Holland to perform the KLAL stem cell surgery on her right eye. Michelle's surgery was December 8, 2004. After two weeks, her eye became very inflamed, so Dr. Holland increased her medication to every thirty minutes. Michelle's medication has been decreased and her right eye is doing well. Presently, she has cataracts, glaucoma, nystagmus, and corneal pannus, with 20/200 (left eye) and 20/400 (right eye) vision. Michelle is a licensed paramedic and works in a nursing home. Also, she has sung a duet with country music star Linda Davis on the The Nashville Network. And she continues to be recertified to drive annually.

On September 25, 1997, Michelle and her husband, Nate, were blessed with a beautiful baby girl, Brianna. During Brianna's examination after birth, she was diagnosed with aniridia. In the fall of 1998, Brianna and her parents were referred to a Vanderbilt University pediatric ophthalmologist. He indicated that Brianna did not have and probably would not develop nystagmus. In addition, he indicated that Brianna's eyesight was much better than Michelle's. Brianna's eyesight is 20/60 and 20/80 in her eyes.

Now, at the age of seven, Brianna is mainstreamed in a regular classroom with only weekly visits with the itinerant teacher for the visually impaired. Brianna does have problems with depth perception and her peripheral vision. Other than that, she functions well. She has played soccer and basketball, and hopes to play softball this spring. In addition, she's taking guitar lessons, enjoys being a cheerleader, and is on the honor roll.

KAREN, U.S.A.—THE IMPORTANCE OF KNOWLEDGE (CHILD WITH WAGR SYNDROME)

At four months old, Kaitlyn was diagnosed. Her pediatrician didn't see anything wrong with her eyes. When I inquired about seeing an eye doctor, the pediatrician wanted to send Kaitlyn to a neurologist first. I said no, I wanted an eye doctor, so that is where we went. When she was diagnosed, I was shocked and disappointed that my daughter wouldn't be able to see things clearly. I was not informed of all the problems associated with aniridia. All I was really told was that she had cataracts and would be light-sensitive. I feel like we fell through the cracks along the way. This should have been diagnosed before she was discharged from the hospital after birth.

Now I have become better educated about it. When she was diagnosed, the Internet really only contained medical literature directed towards doctors. While I understood some of it, most of it was medical terms. Now I feel acceptance of the diagnosis, and my focus is on keeping her vision as healthy as I possibly can.

Kaitlyn was born with cataracts in both eyes. She has not required surgery for them and they have not really grown. She also has nystagmus. Within the last year she has developed glaucoma and is on Cosopt eye drops.

It is important for parents to know to get genetic testing done right away, and then make sure you get the correct results and diagnosis as soon as possible. Kaitlyn was diagnosed with aniridia at four months old. We did take her for her genetic testing shortly thereafter. We took her to a major children's hospital in a big city. They tested her, my husband, and me. They did a good job telling us that we weren't carriers and would have a better chance of winning the lottery while being struck by lightening than having another child with aniridia. They told us that she had a chromosome deletion; to get ultrasounds of her kidneys every three months; and to continue seeing her ophthalmologist. That was it. I had read briefly about WAGR syndrome on the Internet, but in 1997 the only information available was in doctor's terminology that was hard for me to understand. All I understood was what the letters stood for, and I said, "Thank goodness she doesn't have WAGR syndrome." If she'd had WAGR syndrome, the genetics doctor would have told us. She did develop Wilms' tumor at two years, seven months old. Even with the surgery, recovery, and chemotherapy, I still felt lucky that she didn't have WAGR syndrome.

Fast-forward to October 2003. I was looking around the Internet for information on aniridia and nystagmus to print out and give to her teacher. I found Aniridia Foundation International and the Aniridia Network U.K. I joined both sites and introduced myself. The director of the U.K. site wrote me off the list, asking me about Kaitlyn's specific chromosome deletion information. I replied to her with what my letter from the genetic doctor said, and she informed me that my daughter did indeed have WAGR syndrome. That was just as hard to hear and just as heartbreaking as the original diagnosis of aniridia. I felt all the same emotions and then some. It was like being hit with a ton of bricks. I went through the shock, then the anger, before the acceptance. Why was I not told of this? I was given a chromosome deletion sequence, but not given what that chromosome deletion signified. I trusted what the doctor at that hospital told me. It was a major children's hospital in a big city, after all. Five simple words were not spoken by that doctor or written in the letter we received. "Your daughter has WAGR syndrome." Granted, WAGR is very rare, but it is a genetic doctor's job to know about these things. If they aren't sure of what something is exactly, they need to research it further and tell the parents everything they can. So, to wrap this up, my number-one piece of advice for the parents of a newly diagnosed child with aniridia is to get all of the results from the genetic testing and ask one simple question: "Does my child have WAGR syndrome?"

Now Kaitlyn is doing well. First she was in a private school and wasn't eligible to receive many services. At her IEP meetings in first and second grade, they didn't offer much more help than if she went to the public school. Then they offered a significant amount of minutes of care if we would switch her over to public school, so we did. Now that she is in public school; she is enjoying it and gets a lot of services from her vision teacher and orientation and mobility teacher. She gets 300 minutes a week (sixty per day) with her vision teacher and 120 minutes a week (forty minutes every three days) with her orientation and mobility teacher. The O&M takes her out of school and to practical places such as the public library and the post office. In class she sits in the front row and is allowed to approach the dry-erase board when she needs to do so. She is learning to use her monocular. They gave her two desks. One is for sitting and working at, and her school supplies are inside of it. The other is for putting her big, enlarged print textbooks on when in use and storing them when not in use. She didn't have this at the private school and had a hard time with such a small workspace. She just got a CCTV in the classroom and is working on learning to use that. Kaitlyn has always liked to do artwork. It has taken her a while to learn to do simple things like color in the lines and cut out shapes (still choppy-looking), but she is very proud of her completed artwork and loves to show it off, no matter how big or small.

Kaitlyn has a great personality and interacts very well with others. I always get compliments on her attitude and behavior. She is considerate, caring, very polite, and everyone enjoys being around her. She doesn't feel any self-pity and has hardly ever complained about her aniridia. The only times she would say that she wished she had different eyes was each time a sibling was born. My husband and I and the other three kids all have blue eyes. When each sibling came along, she would say that she wishes she had blue eyes, too. After that, she lets it go and really never complains.

JUDY, U.S.A.—GIVEN TO US FOR A REASON

The first time I looked into Jessica's eyes was that mother/child instant-bonding time where every mother knows she is holding the most beautiful baby in the universe. Despite my bliss, I remember thinking that her eyes looked different. They were very dark with just a halo of blue. I naturally assumed she would have blue eyes, since both my husband and I do. When I asked the pediatrician, his response was, "All babies' eyes are dark." Looking back, though, I think my heart knew different.

She was so tiny, weighing only four pounds, fourteen ounces at birth. She was supposed to be born in July, but an ultrasound showed low weight, so our doctor decided that since it would be a Caesarian birth, we would wait until the first week in August, hoping her weight would increase. After her delivery, they discovered the placenta had separated and compromised the normal weight gain during the last month.

She was our tiny bundle of little girl, our joy, and her brother's baby sister. I knew immediately she would wrap her father and me around her little finger, and she did. We have a picture of her dad holding her in the hospital. The camera caught that instant connection that fathers and daughters make right from the start. I couldn't wait to get her home to start our life journey. She was so tiny, though, that the hospital wouldn't let us leave until she reached five pounds.

When we did get home, regular cloth diapers were way too big. We had to use preemie Pampers. Regular baby clothes wouldn't work either, so my mother-in-law made sleepers out of doll clothes patterns. I am still amazed when I see them today and remember how delicate she was then. Everywhere we went, people would stop us and admire her.

At her one-month checkup, the doctor seemed to spend a long time looking at her eyes. When he finished, he said, "I think we need to have an optometrist look at her eyes." When I asked him why, he didn't really answer me. He made an appointment with a local doctor, but we had to wait over two weeks to see him. I was worried. During those two weeks, when I held things in front of her, I wondered if she was seeing them clearly. I thought her irises were stuck open for some reason and wondered what that meant.

When we saw the eye doctor, he darkened the room and spent a long time on the exam. He told us he had never seen a condition like this and that we should see a specialist. He gave us the idea that whatever it was, it could probably be fixed, and made an appointment with two doctors at Riley Children's Hospital in Indianapolis. I felt great hope and knew that the right doctors would know what to do.

It seemed like forever waiting to go to Indianapolis. It was a long trip down there, one that (although we didn't know it at the time) would be repeated several times over the next six years. We went on Election Day in November 1976. She was three months old. I remember this because I was thinking about which candidate I would vote for when we got back home. We had to leave at 4:00 a.m. to make the appointment.

I liked the doctor immediately. He was soft-spoken, kind, and totally involved with Jessica's examination. He looked in her eyes and then spun a black and white cylinder in front of her. It wasn't very long before he was ready to talk. He told us she had congenital aniridia and horizontal nystagmus, and asked if it was in either of our families. He seemed surprised that it was not in either of our families, because it is usually inherited, but in rare instances it just happens. We were full of the ordinary questions: What is it? What caused it? And most importantly, how can we fix it? I remember him saying there was no fix, since it was genetic, and it wasn't something they had a shot or operation for that would make the iris work. The halo of blue would be the only iris she would ever have. I don't recall all of what he said because my mind had to wrap itself around the fact that it wasn't fixable.

I asked him if I could give her one of my eyes. I think he took my hand when he said no. He did smile though and say if transplants were possible there wouldn't be so many visually impaired people, and explained that once the optic nerve was severed it could not be reattached. He went on to tell us that he wanted to do a more thorough exam under anesthetic, and that she should have a kidney x-ray to look for Wilms' tumor. The possibility of a malignant kidney tumor was the hardest news to take, and for the first time I felt scared.

Before we left, I asked where we could get more information about aniridia. At the time, there was not much more than a definition of the condition. This was way before the Internet and easy access to medical information. We made the appointments and started for home. Up until then, I hadn't cried.

The trip home was hard. I remember staring at the utility poles that went by the outside of the car window. I stared at them and cried. I kept trying to figure out how to tell our parents about all we had learned. I did decide not to tell them about the Wilms' tumor possibility. I remember thinking, I'm not strong enough for this, and that she deserves a better mom. I blamed myself over and over for what had happened. I wondered if her low birth weight had anything to do with it. It was a long trip home, and I really don't think Eric and I talked much. Maybe we were both in our own way coming to grips with the news. I nursed her and did all the normal things, but I didn't feel normal.

When we got home, we had planned to vote but didn't. At the time it didn't seem important. Our next appointment was in about a month, and I spent a lot of time writing down questions and trying to find information about aniridia. The best information I found was that the state of Michigan had support for children with special needs. Within a week of my first call, a vision consultant and occupational therapist began making regular visits to our home, and worked out goals and strategies to keep Jessica's development on track. They provided, not only toys and activities, but also friendship and guidance.

Early education and help for parents is really important for low-vision children. In the six years that we continued to go to Indianapolis, we saw lots of children who did not get services until age three or four. There was a definite difference in development. Some of the children we saw would not talk to people, preferred to sit alone, rock back and forth or sway, and did not try to use the vision they had. As a parent, I will forever be grateful for those early years of educational support.

While writing this and looking back over the last thirty years, I have lots of memories about eye doctors, contacts, x-rays, fears, triumphs, and joys. Our journey has involved many supportive people. Some teachers and friends have said what a wonderful job we have done as parents. My response has always been, we didn't do anything special . . . . Jessica did.

ADAM AND JENNIFER, U.S.A. — TYLER'S BETTER TOMORROW

When our son Tyler was first diagnosed with sporadic bilateral aniridia at three months old in June 2003, we were completely taken by surprise. Our pediatrician had previously examined our baby on at least two occasions, going through the motions of checking his pupil dilation as part of a normal wellness exam. In retrospect, we now know that this man could not have been paying adequate attention, because if he had, he would have noticed that there was no pupil dilation, as Tyler did not have an iris in either of his eyes.

We found ourselves unlucky a second time in our pursuit of good medical care: the physician who diagnosed our son was as thoughtless as humanly possible in his handling of the initial, shocking blow. Imagine being told, as new parents, that your son has this "extremely rare" disease and that we should be thankful because "blind people born with their affliction [as opposed to those who become blind later in life] are less likely to go on to commit suicide." After listening to him fumble with Stevie Wonder references in an effort to stop the waterworks from flowing out of my wife's eyes, we finally left this man's office in search of our own answers.

The range of emotions that we experienced was a nonstop back-and-forth between anger and despair. Fear also overwhelmed each of our days, as aniridia was so complex and multifaceted. Would our baby be blind? Would he grow a Wilms' tumor? Should we level with our extended family, or protect them from their own imaginations of what the future would hold? So many thoughts kept us up at night. It was as if a storm had been permanently moored above our home.

There was one break in the clouds during those first few weeks of living with this new life sentence, and her name was Jill Nerby. We first met Jill through countless hours on the phone after having learned of her work with what was then called the U.S.A. Aniridia Network. Before Jill, it seemed to us that our mounting list of questions would forever go unanswered. This misconception would soon be laid to rest, as would the burden of our fear. Many times, Jill would resist the urge to answer our questions herself, instead opting to forward our query to one of the leading experts in each field. It soon became clear to us that this compassionate and devoted woman was more than just a source of comfort to whom parents of newly diagnosed children could turn; she was also enormously well-connected in the medical community, having spent the better portion of her adult life working to decipher who was the best of the best. Through Jill, we had the pleasure of meeting two of the finest physicians in their fields, Dr. Edward Holland and Dr. Peter Netland. We were also fortunate to meet Dr. Sherwin Isenberg, who is now our son's pediatric ophthalmologist.

Almost four years have past since Tyler's diagnosis. We have watched our son grow into an incredibly energetic and remarkably coordinated little boy with highly functional vision. We take him for regular ultrasounds to monitor his kidneys for Wilms', and work hard to comply with the need for regular checkups on his eyes with Dr. Isenberg. Fear has a funny way of subsiding, like a storm that was never predicted and moves out just as fast as it came in, and time is an equal partner in the healing process. We cannot know what the future will hold for our son. All we can do is be grateful for the progress he has made, the care we have received, and the organization formed by Jill Nerby, which to us represents the vessel of hope for Tyler's better tomorrow.

10

Parents' and Families' Guide

JESSICA J. OTIS AND JAMES D. LAUDERDALE

When your child is first diagnosed with aniridia or WAGR syndrome, you will have several questions for your child's ophthalmologist. To be prepared for the first appointment, the best thing to do is make a list of questions. Some questions other parents have had are listed at the end of this chapter. If you choose to, you can use these as a starting point and add more questions to the list as you think of them. At the appointment, be sure to have your list of questions to ask the doctor. Be sure to repeat what the doctor has told you to make sure you understand him or her. If you're not sure, then ask the doctor to try to explain it in a different way so you can understand. It is your child, and you should be as informed as possible, and the only way to do that is to ask questions and to have a good relationship with your child's ophthalmologist.

Other questions parents have had that you do not necessarily need to ask an ophthalmologist will be discussed in this chapter. When a child is first diagnosed, a question asked by many parents, especially mothers, is, "Was this my fault?" No, it was not. Do not ever blame yourself for your child having aniridia or WAGR syndrome. It is a genetic disorder that you could not have done anything about, unless you do have it yourself. There is no reason for you to feel guilty or to put blame on yourself for something you had no control over. One way to help get over any of these feelings is to join Aniridia Foundation International, where you can meet many other parents and people with aniridia. From meeting and speaking with them, you can get the support you need. On AFI's members' area website, I asked parents, "What questions did you have when your child was diagnosed?" One mother responded, "Mainly I wish someone had told us that he would be able to see at least a little bit and that the disastrous picture that was painted for us at the start was not actually representative of what he would turn out to be."

A major question many parents have is, "What is my child's visual acuity, or is my child blind?" Today there is a test that can be done under anesthesia to find out a child's acuity; however, you *must keep in mind* that the first five months of a child's life are crucial to developing long-term vision acuity. The test is called a

142

VEP test, and there are two that can be done on infants and children. They are called "flash and sweep tests." The test will show the brain's response to stimuli, which will help determine what kind of acuity the child has at the time.

A typical question that can follow is, "What does the world look like to him?" This is a very difficult and complicated question to answer. Since aniridia cases can vary, one person may see better than another even though they both have aniridia. Some people with aniridia describe it as like looking through wax paper; however, it must be kept in mind that not everyone with aniridia would describe seeing this way. One way I myself have described it is that I see what you see, just a little blurrier, plus not being able to see things at distances. So as your child grows up and is able to communicate with you, ask him or her to try to describe what he or she sees. It will be the best way for you to understand what the world looks like to him or her.

Another question some parents ask is, "Does nystagmus make my child feel dizzy or uneasy?" Having nystagmus, I can say, absolutely not. Nystagmus has never made me feel dizzy or uneasy. The only time I even somewhat notice the side-to-side movement from it is when I have numbing drops to have my pressure checked, or if I'm very tired. Nystagmus can be more noticeable with some people when they are tired, upset, or nervous.

Other questions you may have:

- Will my child be able to read, or will he or she need to learn Braille?
- Will he or she ever ride a bike?
- Will he or she need a guide dog or white cane to get around?
- What career will he or she be able to have?
- Will he or she be able to have a "normal" life, with friends, maybe a husband or wife, and children of his/her own?
- Will she go to a mainstream school?
- Will our son be able to have children without passing on aniridia?

Regarding the first question, it all depends on the child's visual acuity and whether his/her teacher of the visually impaired (VI teacher) feels learning Braille is necessary. On a personal note, I've never learned Braille and read just fine. I've always been and still am an avid reader of books. Yet it never hurts to learn something that you may need to use in the future. I have thought about learning it just in case.

Riding a bike will also depend on the child's balance and depth perception. As a child, I did learn to ride a bike. I was okay at it, but never felt quite comfortable enough to ride a bike often—but that is just me, it can be different for others. A child with aniridia should be given the chance to learn to ride a bike if he or she wants to learn.

Will your child need a guide dog or white cane to get around? Again, it will depend on the child's visual acuity and depth perception. Curbs and stairs that do not have edges painted can be difficult to see and cause problems for a person with aniridia. Your child's mobility teacher will be the person to ask if he or she thinks your child needs to use a guide dog or white cane.

Will he be able to go to mainstream public school? Most people with aniridia do go to public school and do just fine. Plus, it is important to remember that in the United States the Individual Education Plan (IEP) is available for your child and it can help with their education.

What career will he or she be able to have and will he or she be able to have a "normal" life? To answer the second part of the question, yes. Many people with aniridia live "normal" lives and are married with children and have friends. As far as careers, it can depend on the person's interests and strengths. A person can achieve whatever he or she works hard to do. Many individuals with aniridia have succeeded in the careers of their choice. There are individuals with aniridia who are lawyers, business owners, Olympic gold medallists, pediatricians, and physical therapists.

Will my child be able to have children *without* passing on aniridia? Currently, the medical technology exists to greatly reduce the incidence of passing aniridia from parent to child. However, widespread use of this technology has not been employed in patients afflicted with this disorder.

A person with aniridia normally has a 50 percent chance of passing on aniridia to his/her children, but this percentage can be reduced through the use of genetic screening. Aniridia is caused by mutations that affect one of the two copies of the PAX6 gene, and these mutations can occur in hundreds of different places within the gene. If the *precise* location of the PAX6 mutation is known for the parent, then *preimplantation genetic diagnosis (PGD)* can be used to have children without passing on aniridia. Preimplantation genetic diagnosis is the process of screening embryos for genetic diseases during in vitro fertilization (IVF), and it has been used for more than a decade to screen for hereditary diseases such as Down syndrome and other abnormalities. However, it has not been widely used for aniridia because relatively few parents have been screened to determine the location of their mutation. As more parents learn the location of their mutation, then the use of genetic screening (PGD) to avoid passing aniridia from parent to child can become more common.

PGD is a complicated but highly reliable procedure. In this procedure, an egg and a sperm are combined in a laboratory dish in a process known as IVF. IVF is usually performed on several sets of eggs and sperm to create multiple embryos. When the IVF procedure is successful, the fertilized egg begins to grow by dividing to make more cells. The first division creates a two-cell embryo, both of these cells divide to create a four-cell embryo, and these cells all divide to give an eight-cell embryo. In PGD, one cell from the eight-cell embryo is extracted and examined for chromosomal defects. The removal of a single cell from the eight-cell embryo does not hurt the developing embryo at all. Embryos that do not carry the genetic disorder are then placed back into the mother's uterus to implant and develop naturally. Although PGD is highly reliable, there is a slight chance that embryos carrying a PAX6 mutation will be misdiagnosed and therefore there is still a slight chance of having a child with aniridia. Also, even though the embryos are placed back into the mother's uterus, there is a chance that they might not implant, so the process may have to be repeated.

In summary, genetic screening (PGD) can be used to reduce the incidence of passing aniridia from parent to child, but it can only be performed if the *exact location* of the PAX6 mutation is known in the parent. Although the methods for determining PAX6 mutations are well established, there are very few clinics that will perform such a screening. An increase in the availability of genetic screening for PAX6 mutations will be necessary for more widespread use of PGD. Finally, one may feel that doing PGD is similar to abortion since embryos will be disposed of or have research done on them if they have the PAX6 mutations. Depending on your beliefs and morals, you may choose whether you want to do the test or not.

As mentioned before, you are going through a great deal adjusting to your child's diagnoses. When we are struggling or need support, we often turn to those closest to us, such as family and friends. If someone is a good friend, or especially if he or she is a family member, he or she should want to help you and your child during this time. For them to understand more about your child's condition, you need to sit them down and explain what aniridia is and what may go along with it in the years to come. Explain to them what your child may and may not be able to do, but do not focus too much on the negative aspects. Just make sure to tell them your child should be able to do almost everything that anyone else can do, with a few small exceptions such as driving, seeing long distances, and so on. Having friends and family speak with your child's ophthalmologist or come to an Aniridia Foundation International medical conference may help them understand more.

You will sometimes need to explain aniridia to others in the general public. These types of situations are not always easy to handle, but if you know what you are going to say, then you'll at least know that you tried your best to explain it. You need to know how to explain aniridia in a way that the general public will understand. For example, a stranger asks you why your child looks so sleepy, or why his eyes are moving from side to side. You could say something like, "He has a genetic eye disease called aniridia along with nystagmus. Aniridia causes him to be sensitive to light and glare, and so the eyes protect themselves by being droopy to keep out light, hence the sleepy-eye look. The movement of the eyes is from the nystagmus, because the eyes are trying to find a spot on the retina to have a clear picture." It is up to you how much detail you go into, but just make sure the person understands.

Along with telling people what aniridia is, you could also give examples of what your child can or cannot see. Allow people to ask questions to make sure they understand you correctly. Most people should begin to understand. If not, it might be helpful to give them a brochure on aniridia from Aniridia Foundation International or to tell them to visit Aniridia Foundation International online for the best information, since not all websites on the Internet will have the most up-to-date or correct information on aniridia. One important thing to remember to point out to others is to not take all information on the Internet as the absolute truth. Information on the Internet can be very broad and may not apply to all aniridia cases.

Some misconceptions you may need to be aware of so you can make others aware are:

- Sitting close to a properly functioning television *will not* harm vision.
- Glasses *don't always help* correct limited vision. Some individuals with aniridia do not benefit from corrective lens, but there are some who benefit to some degree.

- Dim lighting *will not* harm the eyes. Actually, most individuals with aniridia require dim lighting to feel more comfortable.
- Holding a book close to one's eyes *will not* harm the eyes.
- Loss of vision in one eye *does not* reduce vision by 50 percent.

One of the first things you should do when your child is diagnosed with aniridia is to check with your state Department of Education to see when your child can begin to receive services. In most states the services begin at birth. When your child enters school it is *very important* to be involved with your child's Individual Education Plan (IEP). Make sure to attend all meetings with your child's school administrator, teacher, and VI teacher to make sure the IEP covers your child's education goals and needs. The IEP is a written plan that includes the child's present level of education performance, annual goals for the child including short-term goals, specific education services to be provided for the child, duration of services, set objectives, set criteria and evaluation procedures, and a scheduled annual evaluation to see if goals are being met. The IEP is crucial to quality education for your child with aniridia. Plus, it is vital for you to know the legal importance of an IEP meeting. At the end of the meeting you will be asked to sign the IEP; however, all parties involved in your child's education should attend the IEP meetings. If a person is absent, you do have the right to meet with the absent person and discuss the IEP before you sign it. Be sure you are an active advocate for your child, and make sure the IEP covers your child's needs.

As your child gets older, you will begin to have other questions about how to deal with certain situations or problems. Some of them could be chores, sports, driving, dealing with bullies, self-esteem, dating, possible eye surgeries, and finding employment.

Chores should be the same for everyone in the household. If you treat a person with aniridia differently from everyone else, he or she will feel different and possibly like less of a person. Just keep in mind that a person with aniridia may do a task differently than someone else might do it. An example could be vacuuming. A person with aniridia may go over the same spot a few times to make sure the carpet is getting vacuumed, since he or she may not be able to see fine details like dirt or sand on the carpet. Although some people with aniridia may use their vision as a way to get out of other things they do not want to do, aniridia *should not* be used as an excuse.

As stated before, you should not treat your child any differently, within reason, than others of the same age. If your child wants to try a sport, you should let him or her try it. Yes, your child might have trouble playing baseball or volleyball because he can't see where the ball is coming from and is not able to react quick enough, but he should at least be given the opportunity to try. It may turn out that he does not like it, or that he really does want to play but feels he is not good enough. This is where you should sit down with the child and tell him that not everyone is good at everything. There are different levels of skills, and he might just have to find the right group of people to play with or the right level of play. Let him know that even professional athletes can make mistakes sometimes, just like everyone else. Also, make sure the child knows that playing a game or a sport should be more about having fun than how good you are at it. If you start telling your child this when he is young, then when he gets older it really should not matter if he is not as good as some of his peers.

A major concern teenagers with aniridia have is dealing with not driving. Make sure you let your teen know that although she cannot drive, she will be able to get wherever she needs to go. Be sure to be available whenever something important is going on for her, so she will not feel left out; however, if you know you will not be home to take her somewhere, try to make other arrangements with a family member or neighbor. If she needs to do something that is not a scheduled event, or it is something that can wait until a little later in time, explain to her that she will get to where she needs to be, just not at that very moment. Make sure she understands that she will not miss anything. Especially be sure to keep your promises, or trust will become a whole other issue. Some teens may feel left out or that they don't have a life because they cannot drive places like their peers, so be sure your teen knows she can still have a good life even though she does not drive. One way to show this could be to have your teen speak with an adult who has aniridia and to even get to know other teens with aniridia, so she can have someone to talk to who understands how she feels.

For some children, a tough situation might be dealing with bullies in school. One of the first things a child needs to know is that if he is being bullied, he should not be afraid or embarrassed to tell someone about it. The next thing he should know is that he needs to walk away. Explain to your child that the "bully" is trying to get a reaction out of him, and if the bully doesn't get a reaction, he will get bored with his game fairly quickly. Also, remind the child that *it's not his or her fault* if he or she is being bullied or teased, especially since most children are bullied or teased at one time or another.

Another major issue may be self-esteem and how to keep it high. When stress is high, we tend to have distorted thinking. For example, a person with aniridia might think, "I have no life because I can't drive. My friends are so lucky!" As a parent we need to help the child or teen to have positive thinking instead, and say, "It's difficult not being able to drive and have the freedom that all my friends do, but I have really great friends and family who take me where I need to go." Try to always be positive in front of your child. Children learn many negative thoughts and behaviors from their role models. In addition, it is a good idea to give your child positive reinforcement. Do not always tell her what she is doing wrong or how she could do something better. Find something that she does well and let her know. This will make her feel good about herself, and she will begin to feel worth something. Let your child know that aniridia or WAGR syndrome is only one part of her, and there are many great things about her. Do not make unrealistic comparisons. For example, if your child tells you his brother who has no visual impairment can hit a softball better than he can, explain to him that it is easier for his sibling to see the ball, and therefore he is able to hit it easier. Don't make your children feel as though it is one against the other and they have to see who can do something better. Just tell them that there are some things that one person is good at while there are other things that the other person can do better. Also, make sure he is not getting upset that someone else can finish reading or doing something faster than he can. It would obviously be unrealistic for someone with a visual impairment to be able to read just as fast as someone with 20/20 vision. Do not over-generalize. Let your child know that if there is something he cannot do as a result of his disability, it is not fair to conclude that he is an overall failure. Help your child to avoid getting caught using "should" statements such as "I should be able to finish this chapter in ten minutes just like the rest of the class."

As your child gets older, he or she will want to date. For someone with aniridia, it can be difficult to meet someone to date for a few reasons. It can be difficult to see someone's expression from across a room. Also, some people may not be open-minded and not be interested because the person with aniridia may look tired or drunk because of ptosis. Plus, since the war on drugs, many people do not want to be associated with someone who has drug or alcohol problems. However, both these problems can be solved. For example, your child is in college and goes to a party. She can see an attractive man across the room. But she cannot see that he is making eye contact and smiling at her, so she does not smile back. He thinks she is not interested and does not approach her. Instead of expecting him to approach her, she may need to be more outgoing and approach him on her own so he can see she is interested. In dealing with those who are not open-minded, she will need to be confident and comfortable with explaining aniridia and ptosis to those who ask or notice her eyes. Only in this way will the man understand why she looks tired. Also, a way to meet others would be to get involved in groups or clubs, which will allow people to get to know the person with aniridia first and not judge them on their physical appearance before they know the person.

A very stressful situation some children, teenagers, and young adults may have to go through is eye surgeries for glaucoma or stem cells and cornea transplants. This process will be a very difficult experience for your child, and for you as a parent to see your child go through it. To help your child during the process, you can call and see if you can get a tour of the hospital or facility to help you both feel more comfortable in the environment. When your child asks you a question, try to be as positive and honest as possible, but not overly detailed, and speak to him or her on his/her level so the child understands. Let your child pack his or her suitcase to help him or her feel more in control of the situation, and let the child bring a stuffed animal or blanket that may help him or her feel more secure. Before the surgery you may also want to use play therapy or role-playing with a stuffed animal to help your child express his/her feelings. These techniques can help a child express his/her fears or concerns about the surgery that he or she may not tell you without the stuffed animal speaking for him or her. Some other suggestions are: talking to the child in a soft soothing voice, having soft soothing music playing while preparing for the surgery, and allowing the child to draw to express his or her feelings. Lastly, ask if you can accompany your child into the operating room. If it is not possible, try to stay with your child for as long as possible, and then see your child in recovery as soon as you are allowed to do so.

For teenagers and young adults, the most you can do is encourage them to express their feelings in a way that is good for them. Some things teenagers or young adults may fear are loss of control and going under anesthesia. To help your teen or young adult feel more in control, allow him or her to be a part of decision-making during the process. Offer support during the procedure, but if he or she wants more independence, take a step back so not to make him or her uncomfortable. For more information on how to help your child through the experience of surgery, go to http://www.cincinnatichildrens.org/svc/alpha/c/child-life/families/hospitalization/tips.htm or http://www.pana.org/childreninsurgery.htm.

When your child becomes a teenager or young adult, he or she may discover getting a job can be difficult. Finding and getting hired for a job is a job within itself; however, there are services in each state that can help a visually impaired individual find employment. Please keep in mind that the services in each state can vary. To find out what type of services your state provides, please visit http://www.ilru.org/html/publications/directory/index.html. This link will take you to a national listing of Centers for Independent Living. All you have to do is click on your state, and it will take you to your state's list. Another website that may be helpful in your child's job search is the Office of Disability Employment (U.S. Department of Labor). To visit this website, go to http://www.dol.gov/odep/. For more information on other resources, please visit http://www.hicom.net/%7Eoedipus/blind.html.

In conclusion, as parents we want the best for our children, but sometimes life deals them a difficult hand. So we need to help them through by supporting them as much as possible. Allow your child to explore and try new things. You never know, he or she may surprise you with how much he or she can do.

QUESTIONS FROM OTHER PARENTS THAT YOU MIGHT ASK YOUR DOCTOR

- How did he or she get aniridia?
- Who can do a VEP test to determine his/her vision acuity?
- Should we get genetic testing done? Where?
- Is there anything we can do to protect his/her eyes to help prevent other things such as glaucoma, cataracts, etc.?
- Where can we get infant/child sunglasses and what darkness/color lenses should we get?
- What should we expect during an appointment to check his or her pressure or ultrasound for Wilms' tumor when he or she is under anesthesia?
- Since he or she has familial aniridia, should he or she still be tested for Wilms' tumor?
- How is cancer of the kidneys associated with aniridia?
- What is the Wilms' tumor risk factor for someone with aniridia?
- Can anything be done medically to improve his vision or photophobia?
- Will the cataracts grow larger?
- Will wearing glasses correct low vision associated with aniridia?
- After the initial diagnosis, should anything be done to stimulate the baby/child to use his eyes, and if so, what?
- Should an ultrasound be carried out every three months even though your child does not have WAGR?

- What limitations/challenges may he face in childhood and later on?
- Is anybody researching aniridia?
- Is there any way we can recognize the signs of glaucoma starting?
- If we have more children, will they also have aniridia?
- What technology is available for this?
- How often should my child have eye exams and pressure checks?
- What kind of medical progress is being made to help this condition in the future?

11

Teachers' and School Administrators' Guide

JILL ANN NERBY AND JESSICA J. OTIS

A child with aniridia is being placed in your classroom, and you may be wondering whether their needs are different from those of your other students. This information has been written to answer any questions or concerns about this new teaching experience.

When a child with a visual disability is enrolled in a regular class, careful consideration is given to assess whether he or she can compete both academically and socially. Although he or she may need to cope with visual and emotional stresses usually not encountered by non-disabled children, he or she will soon become a fully participating member of the class.

In order to ensure that the child with aniridia has the opportunity to reach their full academic potential, the child and you will hopefully receive the supportive services of a special teacher of the visually impaired (VI teacher) to discuss classroom situations. A child with aniridia is generally considered eligible for special services of a resource and/or VI teacher if their measured visual acuity is 20/70 or less in the better eye with corrective lenses (in other words, if what he or she can see at twenty feet is no more than what a person with normal vision sees at seventy feet). Children who have a measured visual acuity of 20/200 or less in the better/corrected eye or who have a visual field of no greater than twenty degrees are classified as legally blind.

WHAT IS ANIRIDIA?

Aniridia is a partial or complete absence of the iris, and it may be associated with other ocular defects such as macular and optic nerve hypoplasia, cataract, corneal surface abnormalities that lead to decreased vision, and nystagmus. The vision may fluctuate, depending on lighting conditions and glare. Glaucoma is a secondary problem causing additional visual loss over time. Because of poor visual acuity and nystagmus, low-vision aids are very helpful. Lifelong regular follow-up care is necessary for early detection of any new problem so that timely treatment is given. If a person has a cataract, this is a condition in which the normally transparent lens of the eye becomes cloudy or opaque. *Glaucoma* is a condition in which pressure of the fluid inside the eye is too high. Depending upon the type of glaucoma, visual loss may be gradual, sudden, or present at birth. *Nystagmus* is a rapid movement of the eyeballs from side to side, up and down, in a rotary motion, or a combination of these movements, which the child with aniridia cannot control voluntarily.

For more information, visit Aniridia Foundation International (AFI) online at www.aniridia.net. Please keep in mind that not all websites on the Internet will have the most up-to-date or correct information on aniridia, so one important thing to remember and to point out to others is to not take all information on the Internet as the absolute truth, since information on the Internet can be very broad and may not apply to all aniridia cases.

It is important to remember that visually impaired children differ in their ability to use their vision. Two children may have the same measured acuity, but one may rely on his other senses to perform the same tasks that the other child does by sight. These individual differences *must* be respected.

Another consideration is that aniridia affects the child's visual functioning, and their vision will generally fluctuate slightly from day to day or even throughout a given day. Even stable visual conditions may be temporarily influenced by factors such as lighting, fatigue, and emotions. As the child's classroom teacher, you will soon become sensitive to the individualized needs of your student with aniridia. The older the child is, the better he or she is able to communicate his or her abilities and limitations. You may discuss with the VI teacher the specific needs or limitations related to your student's specific visual disability or disabilities as mentioned in this chapter. You and the VI teacher can work together to provide a happy, stimulating educational experience in which, not only the student with aniridia, but also the entire class will benefit. Recognize each child as a special person! The child with aniridia is a child first, who happens to have a visual disability.

Aniridia and Autism

There have been recent studies showing that a person with aniridia can also have autism. For more up to date information on this, please visit www.aniridia.net.

HOW CAN YOU HELP THE STUDENT WITH ANIRIDIA FEEL COMFORTABLE IN YOUR CLASSROOM?

- Introduce and address the student with aniridia by name as you would any student. Questions will certainly arise from other children and adults. Encourage the child to answer these questions for him/herself.
- Include the student with aniridia in all activities (physical education, home economics, industrial arts, etc.). The VI teacher can offer suggestions about

methods and special equipment or aids that may be helpful in some activities.

- At times all children like to be the center of attention (team captain, line leader, etc.). Encourage the student with aniridia to take leadership positions just like other children do.
- The same disciplinary rules that apply to the rest of the class should apply to the student with aniridia.
- Encourage the child with aniridia to move about the classroom to obtain his materials or visual information. He will know his own needs and method of compensating, and will soon become part of classroom routine.
- The child with aniridia may not be aware of and therefore may not become interested in events occurring at a distance from her, since she may not notice them. Some examples are a facial expression, a nod, and arm or hand movements. All of these could be used to invite a person to come over to you, to respond to a question, or to get an item. However, for a child with aniridia, you will need to use verbal cues. For example: "Jane, on top of the computer in the back of the room, there is a green folder, could you get it for me?"
- If necessary, provide additional work, desk, or locker space as needed to accommodate special materials (bulky large print books, reading stands, or other adaptive aids).
- As you and others get to know the student with aniridia, the other students may become interested in topics related to vision and visual impairment. You may wish to incorporate this into class lessons. If the child with aniridia feels comfortable about this information, he may want to participate in the presentation of the lesson.
- All children are sensitive to peer criticism. Your own acceptance of the child with aniridia will serve as a positive role model for the class. It is very important to educate students and staff members in the school about matters concerning visual disability in order to better manage the behaviors of student "bullies" or negative comments. These comments can have a detrimental impact upon the self-esteem of the child with aniridia and may cause depression in some. Possibly a classroom teacher could implement a "Character Education" program to help students develop positive attitudes towards people with disabilities. A heightened level of knowledge will lead to an increased degree of understanding and to valuing individual differences.
- The student with aniridia may bring adaptive aids into the classroom. Encourage her to use the aids as needed, and to answer any questions that others have about the aids as they arise.
- Because some visually impaired children prefer not to bring attention to their disability, they will use special aids and assistance from others only when absolutely necessary. In general, you should respect the child's wishes, but if you suspect he really needs more aids or assistance than he is using, you may wish to consult with the VI teacher about this matter.

- A child with aniridia will learn to avoid obstacles in the classroom and school corridors. The VI teacher will alert you if there are any specific problems (stairs, outside playground, unmarked curbs, dimly lighted areas, etc.) and how to help the child maneuver these areas safely.
- For the safety of the student with aniridia as well as for all other children, doors and cupboards should be all the way open or all the way shut. She should also be told of any changes in the position of classroom furniture.

WHAT SPECIAL DEVICES WILL THE STUDENT WITH ANIRIDIA USE?

Some children with aniridia may need only a few adaptive materials while others require a combination of several devices. A partial list is below.

Non-optical aids—These are devices that are not individually prescribed, and may or may not be designed specifically for a person with a visual disability.

Visual Aids

- Bookstands may help reduce postural fatigue by bringing the work closer to the reader's eyes. When a bookstand is not available, one may be improvised by placing other books beneath the book the child is reading.
- Felt-tip or dark writing pens provide a darker letter or drawing, and black ink is usually preferred. Using different colored markers or highlighters will often help a student to emphasize sections of their notes when scanning would otherwise be quite difficult.
- Acetate or transparency sheets/clear see-through tinted sheets. A general preference is yellow. Tinted transparencies placed over the printed page will tend to darken the print as well as heighten its contrast with the background of the paper, which lessens the glare.
- Large-print books may provide comfort for those who cannot read regular print at a close distance even with an optical aid. Its quality or typeface is as important to legibility as its size. Spacing between letters and lines is also important.
- There is a type of paper available for those with visual impairments. This paper has dark, bold lines and is helpful to children who find it difficult to see the lines on regular writing paper. Bold lines are available in various formats, such as graph paper and large-print staves for music notation.
- Page markers and reading windows may be helpful to a child who finds it difficult to focus on a word or line of print.
- Since a person with aniridia is sensitive to light and glare, sun visors and other shields may be used in certain situations to block out some of the light and glare. Outside it is normally done with sunglasses and/or brimmed hats.
- Textbook publications may be available in electronic format from the publisher.

- Students with aniridia may benefit from an elevated slope for easier reading. This also helps them avoid poor posture while reading and writing. Ask the child's VI teacher about it. Placing a book on the desk and then leaning the reading book up against it to create a slope can create a homemade version of the slope. This also helps with worksheets and tests.

Auditory Aids

- Cassette tape recorder—Students can use the recorder to take notes, listen to recorded texts, or formulate compositions or writing assignments.
- Cassette players/recorders and other recording programs—The Library of Congress and other organizations provide free library services to people with visual disabilities by offering a wide variety of texts and leisure reading on cassettes, and most recently, CDs. The speeds at which the cassettes and CDs are played differ from the speeds of commercially manufactured recordings; therefore, the Library of Congress lends special cassette players to eligible individuals. Some cassette players provide a variable speed component, which can be adjusted to suit the needs of the listener.

Assistive Technological Aids

- Talking calculator—This hand-held calculator speaks each entry and result. It is capable of performing all the necessary computations, and earphones are available.
- Closed-circuit television (CCTV)—The CCTV enlarges printed materials onto a computer-like monitor, and can also change polarity: black print on a white background on paper can be viewed as white print on a black background (which cuts out a lot of glare). Color contrasts and illumination can also be altered.
- Computerized assistive technology—There are software programs that are capable of enlarging print and graphics on the computer monitor, such as Zoomtext, Bigshot, and Window-Eyes. Ask the VI teacher how to get this technology for your student. There are also dictation programs that allow a person to speak into a microphone, and the computer types what the person says.

Optical Aids

- Glasses with special prescriptions may be prescribed for a child with aniridia if he or she will benefit from the lens correction.
- Tinted lenses—The child with aniridia generally needs to wear tinted glasses inside as well as darker tinted glasses outside.
- Magnifiers will increase the size of the image reaching the eye.

- Bioptic monocular (telescopic aid)—children can use a monocular (hand-held or placed in spectacle frames) to view the chalkboard and class demonstrations.

HOW WILL THE CHILD WITH ANIRIDIA WORK WITH PRINTED MATERIALS?

Chalkboard Notes

- When the chalk or marker board is located in the front of the classroom, the front row, center, is usually a good seat for a child with a visual disability. However, not all front-row seats will guarantee that the child with aniridia will be able to see everything written on the chalkboard. If demonstrations are given during class, the location of the demonstration should be taken into consideration when assigning permanent seats. A child with aniridia will experience glare in certain situations, which may cause her discomfort or inability to read, and she will prefer a seat away from the window or other bright light. It is helpful for the child with aniridia to sit with her back to the sun.
- If he's using a marker board, ask the child with aniridia which color of marker he can see best. Some colors such as red and green are more difficult for some to see. Black or blue are usually preferred most.
- Assign a cooperative classmate to copy or read notes aloud in a low voice to the child with aniridia.
- Encourage the child with aniridia to walk up to or move his chair closer to the chalkboard, and help him to position himself so as not to block the view of other students.
- Lend the student with aniridia your copy of the notes you put on the board or the book from which you have taken them.
- *Say the notes aloud as you are writing them on the board.* The child with aniridia can take them down as dictation.
- Enlarge and darken your notes on a copy machine for the student with aniridia. This is especially helpful in a math class, where following step-by-step instructions is necessary.

Demonstrations in Class

- When you have a student with aniridia, it is best not to stand with your back to the window. Glare and light will silhouette your demonstration and will make it visually uncomfortable for the student with aniridia. Cutting down on glare will benefit the entire class.
- Allow the child with aniridia to stand next to or to the side of the demonstration. Consider allowing her to assist in doing the demonstration or to handle the materials before or after the observation period.
- A CCTV may be useful and permit magnification of the demonstration.

Maps and Charts

- The child with aniridia may wish to move closer to the chart or even sit on the floor (if appropriate). Permit him to do so as long as he does not block another child's view.
- An enlarged copy of the chart or map may be given to the child. Ask the VI teacher if she is able to provide enlarged or otherwise modified available maps. Some maps or diagrams may need to be simplified for ease in viewing.

Movies, Projectors, Reading Machines, and PowerPoint Presentations

- If it is possible for the child with aniridia to preview a movie on a TV monitor, allow him to sit close enough to see it. If there are subtitles, request that another classmate read the titles aloud to the student or class.
- Poor contrast or insufficient lighting with certain reading machines, such as microfiche, may present reading problems for the child with aniridia. Here are a couple of suggestions. Using a clear yellow overlay may help with contrast when she is reading microfiche. Another student with the same assignment could read the material aloud to her if the child with aniridia feels comfortable with it. However, the older the child gets, the more she will just want to "fit in" and not want to draw attention to herself in this way. The individual responsible for audio/visual materials in a school can be a resource for adaptive ideas and devices to be used in the classroom, as can the VI teacher.

Reproduced Materials, Tests, and Homework

Consult with the VI teacher as to the appropriate print size and clarity needed for the student with aniridia. The following suggestions may be helpful when children with visual disabilities find reprints unclear or difficult to read.

- Ask the VI teacher how to adapt or enlarge instructional materials on a copy machine. It is also helpful if you give the student with aniridia the assignments, particularly long-term projects and reports, as far in advance as possible. This will allow for any special ordering of materials or locating human readers.
- He will frequently need extra time to complete assignments and exams. Allowing time and a half is usually considered acceptable. When you are certain the child understands the work, it may be a good idea to shorten his assignments. For example, you may request that he do only the odd-numbered problems in the math homework.
- When making copies of tests or worksheets, be sure the print is large and dark enough for the child with aniridia to read. Black ink is usually easier to read. Do not use red, green, or blue.

- You may use separate answer sheets for students to use while taking a test; however, it is generally easier for a child with a visual disability to answer directly on the test.

Texts and Other Books

Many students with aniridia can use books with regular-size type, although they may have to bring the book closer to their eyes and use optical aids or reading stands. They may also require more time to complete assignments.

- If a child requires or feels more comfortable with large print or recordings, then these may be obtained by the VI teacher for her. If you are aware that you will have a child with aniridia, you may want to give titles of the books to be used to the VI teacher even before the student enters the class. Children who qualify as "legally blind" are entitled to receive from the federal government specialized equipment distributed through the American Printing House for the Blind in Louisville, Kentucky.
- As a child gets older and moves on to high school, more subjects will be offered, such as home economics. In such a class, when doing something like sewing, a visually impaired person may benefit from using contrasting thread colors, such as light thread on dark material or dark thread on light material. For more suggestions on how to help a visually impaired student in this type of class, please ask the student's VI teacher.
- In the upper grades, students often request their own recorded or otherwise adapted texts through organizations such as Recording for the Blind.

HOW WILL THE STUDENT WITH ANIRIDIA MANAGE IN ACTIVITIES OUTSIDE THE CLASSROOM?

A frequent concern of regular classroom teachers is the safety of a student with a visual disability. While certain precautions must sometimes be taken, it is important not to project your own fears onto the child with aniridia. The student's needs for exploration and independence must be balanced with sound safety practices, which often should be enforced for all children. However, the child with a visual impairment should not be excluded from activities in the belief that she might hurt herself, unless restrictions are specified by her physician or ophthalmologist.

On the other hand, some children prefer not to participate in certain activities. A child with aniridia may find it very difficult to participate in ball games in which quick focusing, depth perception, and detail vision are necessary. Again, you may wish to consult with the VI teacher to provide suggestions as to how the student with aniridia may participate in sports in a meaningful way, such as assisting the team's coach or taking score. It may be necessary to find other activities that he can do and get other students involved in a meaningful way. Some of the following suggestions may be helpful around the school, both inside and out. Individuals with aniridia may have good indoor and outdoor travel skills, but may have trouble with depth perception, such as unmarked steps, or unnoticeable small holes or dips on a playground.

- Fire drills—The child with aniridia should be instructed to walk with or take hold of a nearby classmate or adult, and quickly and quietly follow others. Assigning a sighted student is ineffective when the assigned student is absent or panics.
- Auditorium—The child may choose to sit closer to the stage and should be allowed to do so.
- Field trips—When visiting a theater, a museum, or other exhibits, you may want to notify someone on the staff that there is a visually impaired student in your class. If told in advance, they may allow the child with aniridia to go beyond museum barriers or touch some of the exhibits.
- Lunchroom—Initial orientation to the lunchroom may be necessary so that the child learns where the trays are located, where the line forms, etc.

WHAT ADDITIONAL SKILLS, MATERIALS, OR ASSISTANCE DOES THE CHILD WITH A VISUAL IMPAIRMENT RECEIVE FROM A VI TEACHER?

- Listening skills—These skills enable the child with a visual disability to make efficient use of her hearing, and are particularly important for listening to recorded texts and obtaining information from teacher presentations and class discussions. Tuning in to sounds in the environment is also essential for the development of her orientation and mobility skills. Listening skills taught by the VI or mobility teacher can supplement those taught in the regular classroom.
- Daily living skills—These are essential for the development of independence and a feeling of self-worth. They include the "how to's" of daily living, from good grooming, to cooking a simple meal, to organizing and locating belongings.
- Orientation and travel skills—The child will be taught the basics of movement and travel skills as needed by a mobility teacher.
- Visual skills—The VI teacher will help a child with a visual disability to discover the conditions under which he can best use his vision, such as types of illumination, positioning of materials, type size, and so on.
- Materials—Special or adapted materials may be obtained for use in the classroom. The VI teacher will help your student to learn to care for the tools and equipment she uses.

ADDITIONAL ASSISTANCE

- Concept development—The child who has been severely visually impaired since birth may need to be taught the body image and spatial concepts that the sighted child normally develops as a matter of course. For example, a child may need to learn such spatial concepts as "above," "below," and "next to" in relation to himself and others. Older students may have difficulty understanding the concepts of rotation and revolution. The child also needs to learn concrete educational experiences. By using real objects he can learn about the environment around him.

- Remedial academic assistance—The VI teacher may be able to help you locate tutors or otherwise provide for remediation if this should be necessary.
- Counseling and guidance—One of the most important jobs of a teacher is to provide an understanding atmosphere in which the child with a visual disability can express her physical disability. It is necessary to help the child cope with the attitudes of others. With you and other supportive staff, the student will learn to communicate their needs and concerns. The school's guidance department also shares the responsibility of personal counseling and career education. A student with aniridia approaching the age of fourteen should also consult with a vocational counselor from the state agency or department concerned with the needs of the visually impaired. Students with a visual disability should become aware of their state's programs for financial assistance in higher education and vocational planning.

RELATED TOPICS OF INTEREST

- It is important to remember that a young child with aniridia, particularly if the child's vision condition has been stable from birth, may not be aware that what he is seeing is any different from what other children see. A gradual visual loss is also difficult for a child with aniridia to detect and verbalize. For example, the child may not realize that there is increased glaucoma pressure in his eyes.
- It is extremely important that the regular classroom teacher, the VI teacher, parents, and other support service school staff maintain positive open communication for the benefit of the student's success in school. Everyone must work towards helping the student with aniridia to reach their maximum potential in every aspect of life.
- One way to help the student excel and for you to stay connected with the child's parents and VI teacher is to be involved with the child Individual Education Plan (IEP). Make sure the parents understand how important an IEP is and how it can help the child.

Some possible warning symptoms of deterioriating eyesight can be placed in one of the three major groupings listed below.

- Physical changes of or about the eyes and face—These include an eye that tends to wander or eyes that are bloodshot or show recurrent redness or watering. The child may complain that her eye hurts either at various times of the day or during specific tasks. Frequent rubbing of the eyes is another symptom of trouble. Facial distortions, frowning, or an abnormal amount of squinting or blinking are also possible signs of problems. A child may show preference for using only one eye, for viewing at close range, or bring objects unusually close to her eyes.

- Changes in vision—A child may complain that objects look blurry or that he is unable to see something at a relatively close distance. He may have an unusual tendency to hold his hand close to his eyes or move it in front of him. An inability to use vision in different types of situations or illumination should also be noted.
- Changes in behavior—A child may become irritable when doing deskwork or show a short attention span when watching an activity that takes place across the room.

CLEARING UP SOME COMMON MISCONCEPTIONS ABOUT VISION

- Glasses *do not always help* correct limited vision. While some visually limited children will be aided to an extent by corrective lenses, there are many for whom correction is not possible, and many who can benefit somewhat from correction but will still have very limited vision.
- Holding a book close to one's eyes will not harm one's vision. Individuals with aniridia often do this to help compensate for the size of the print.
- If a television is functioning properly, sitting close to the set *will not harm the eyes*.
- Sight *cannot* be conserved. Unless you have been informed otherwise, encourage a child to use their vision.
- Dim light *will not* harm the eyes. As a result of some eye conditions (aniridia, cataracts, albinism), a child may require dim lighting in order to visually feel more comfortable.
- Loss of vision in one eye *does not* reduce vision by 50%. While there is loss of vision on the affected side and a general loss of depth perception, it is not a loss of half the visual system.

For more information about aniridia, please visit the Aniridia Foundation International's (AFI) Physicians and Professionals area by logging on to the website www.aniridia.net. In this area there is a special page for teachers. AFI adds new information on a continual basis, so go there often. If you have any helpful suggestions that have not been printed, please send them to teachers@aniridia.net so that AFI may add them to that area.

12

Jill Nerby and Aniridia Foundation International

JESSICA J. OTIS

Jill Nerby was the first to welcome me to Aniridia Foundation International (AFI) when I joined. Shortly after beginning to volunteer for AFI's members' news-letter, I approached Jill about doing this book. Instantly she approved of my idea and told me if I needed anything to let her know. She has been instrumental in shaping the book's content and eliciting the participation of all the doctors and professionals. Her support and wisdom have helped create this informative book for you, and they have meant a great deal to me. She is caring and friendly to all. Jill inspires us to strive towards goals for AFI and in our own lives. Here is her inspiring personal life story and the tale of how she began Aniridia Foundation International (formally the USA Aniridia Network).

Jill Ann Nerby was born in Milwaukee, Wisconsin, in 1961 to her parents, Dennis and Sullen Nerby. She was officially diagnosed with aniridia when she went for her three-week check-up. Jill's parents were told that she was only the second person in the state of Wisconsin to be diagnosed with aniridia. Dr. George Worm realized something was wrong with her eyes and sent her to a well-known ophthalmologist in Chicago, Illinois, with experience in aniridia. This doctor tested Jill for glaucoma and found that she had been born with it. She was then put on eye drops, since the doctor felt Jill was too young to have surgery. Jill's parents were devastated, since she was their first child and the family's first grandchild. They did not even know if she could see and thought she might be blind already. They asked many people and sisters at the Catholic convent to pray for Jill. Today Jill has a younger sister, Marybeth, and a younger brother, Jeff; they do not have aniridia.

Jill says growing up was challenging at times. Kids would sometimes tease her, leave her out, or pick her last. People with aniridia sometimes have droopy eyelids to help control light, which some people mistake for the person looking sleepy or drunk. Jill distinctly remembers how, one time in first grade, a group of older kids gathered around her at recess, and one boy said, "Hey, look, this little girl is stoned." Jill did not know what "stoned" meant, so the comment did not bother her. What did hurt her was that she'd drawn attention to herself and her eyes. That day after school she ran home to ask her mom what "stoned" meant. Through the years, frequent comments such as this have bothered her because she did not want to be associated with the type of people who do drugs. The comments especially troubled her when she tried to find a job. However, Jill did not seem to have much problem with schoolwork. She adapted and made good grades. Unfortunately, an IEP (Individual Education Plan) and other special devices were not available to her at the time, so she just sat up close to the board and held her book close to her face. Surprisingly, Jill was especially good in reading. In grade school in Wisconsin they used an IGE (Individual Guided Education) plan for everyone. If a student needed more help, she was placed with all the children who were at the same level. If a student excelled, she was with all those who also found it easy. In Jill's third-grade year she was tested and found above-average for her grade level. With the IGE system, each grade had a low, medium, and high-level reading group. Grades one through five had the same classes at the same time. Jill was in the third-grade rooms for every class except reading. For that she was sent to the highest reading class for the fifth graders. This highest reading group was a very small group of boys. Jill was the only girl and a third grader. Jill remembers how they put on a spoof play of the *Wizard of Oz,* and of course she was Dorothy.

In middle school, Jill wore glasses and played flute in the band. She also took organ lessons. For Jill, reading music was difficult from a distance, and she usually had to memorize it. She was also a cheerleader and in the Folk Dancing competition squad.

When Jill moved on to high school, she got contact lenses. She also reunited with the older kids she had been friends with in middle school. She made good grades, belonged to the drama club, and was a wrestling team backer (girlfriends of the wrestlers). Jill's first love was Jim. As freshmen, Jim and Jill were voted runners-up for king and queen for their winter prom. Jill and Jim were high school sweethearts then fifteen years later they had their son, Michael. During high school Jim and Jill also belonged to a competition drum and bugle corps for the city. They played baritone bugle. It required countless of hours practicing, traveling to competitions, parades, and camps that worked them about sixteen hours a day. However, Jill says it was the one of the best times of her life.

In her later high school years, Jill's dad was transferred to Memphis, Tennessee, so needless to say Jill was discontented about it. She often went back to Wisconsin to live during the summers so that she could march with the drum and bugle corps, and to take care of her maternal grandmother, Frances Pagel, who was diagnosed with leukemia in 1977. Jill and her grandmother were *very close*. Jill misses her grandmother dearly and wishes she could have seen that there is now help for those with aniridia.

In school, Jill had a lot of opportunities. She had attained almost all of the credits needed to graduate by her sophomore year, but was lacking the English of junior and senior years. So she took electives such as newspaper staff and psychology. In her junior year, Jill headed up the advertising staff of the school paper, attended a couple of morning classes, was a reporter for the local paper, and started to attend radio and TV courses offered at a different school in the afternoons. Her senior year she went to a couple of classes in the morning, and then went to work at a local radio station in the afternoon, doing a weekly news show. She learned a lot from the news anchor, Alan Loudell. Jill says it was strange being in high school and sort of not being in high school; however, it got her a lot of experience and it was enjoyable to talk to the station's owner, Sam Phillips of Sun Studios and Elvis Presley fame. Jill graduated and went off to college.

Jill's later college years were more challenging because her corneal scarring had increased. She had the Students with Disabilities helping with her adaptations. She sought solutions, but was not impressed with the odds given for a corneal transplant. They said it could be 50 percent better or 50 percent worse than before the surgery. Today we know that there is virtually zero percent chance of success for an individual with aniridia to have a successful corneal transplant, since it does not address the underlying problem of limbal stem cell deficiency. So Jill just went on studying the best she could. She graduated from college with a bachelor of science degree, majoring in psychology and biology. Most of her elective courses were in genetics, and that convinced Jill to go back to college in hopes of going into the medical field. Jill worked at a hospital in the occupational therapy department while taking her pre-med courses, but her vision continued to decline. Jill never made it to occupational therapy school. She soon accepted this as, not a defeat, but a sign that her life and talents were being guided elsewhere.

As Jill's vision started diminishing, she became more and more frustrated with her loss of independence. Jill hated to ask for help and was bound and determined to accomplish things on her own. Jill's frustration increased as she tried to find things about aniridia on the Internet, and found virtually nothing except definitions such as "aniridia: meaning lack of iris." To Jill this was frustrating because she knew there was more to it, and that information was not being put out there for people like her.

Feeling that there just had to be something to help her regain her sight from the corneal scarring, Jill thought if they were using stem cells for breast cancer, why not for eyes? So Jill typed in some medical terms and came up with an article about Dr. Edward Holland experimenting with KLAL surgery on with a person with aniridia. Jill then met Dr. Holland. Once she went to him and he started treating her, Jill realized that *he's really got something here*. Jill later asked him to be on the executive board of directors of Aniridia Foundation International, because of his experience with people with aniridia and corneal disease.

When Jill began her treatment with Dr. Holland, she found more resistance from the insurance companies, who had absolutely no clue why she needed this "experimental transplant." This was again because of lack of education, information, and public awareness. Jill says, "You have never been frustrated and angry until you wait for years for something to restore your sight, then find it, and are told you cannot have it or, should we say, that they will not cover it." Jill had the KLAL done, but since the cornea scarring was so deep in her cornea, she also needed to have a corneal transplant done three months later. The corneal transplant would not have worked if Dr. Holland had not done the KLAL first, since people with aniridia need to have the stem cells first in order for the cornea transplant to work.

Jill was enjoying her new vision that was restored by her first KLAL and cornea transplant while taking care of her paternal grandmother, Jane Nerby, who was diagnosed with peritoneal cancer in May 2001. She was one of Jill's best friends all her life, and they would talk for hours. Her family even says that they were very much alike, with the same actions and mannerisms. One summer Jill had told her grandmother how she wanted to help others find the way to restored sight, educate the public so there would be no more "misconceptions" about those with a visual impairment (especially aniridia), and make things better for the children of today and tomorrow being born with aniridia. "Yet I do not think I can tackle such a big job," Jill told her. Jill's grandmother always uplifted her and told her she could do whatever she put her mind to do.

That is when Jill decided to start the USA Aniridia Network, which has expanded worldwide and is now called Aniridia Foundation International. Jill then met some others with aniridia and told them she wanted to start a support group, but with a definite medical aspect to it. The foundation first came together as an official group at the Memphis medical conference. She has been working on and adding onto it ever since. Jill has had some very dedicated members and doctors helping along the way, and feels that things fell into place because they were meant to be.

Then, with her family surrounding her, Jane Nerby passed away on September 21, 2001. Sadly, Jill's grandmother passed away only three months before the foundation was classified as an official 501(c)3 nonprofit organization. She never got to see the results of her pep talk to Jill. Now Jill, her parents, and her grandfather (Larry Nerby) carry Jane's memory in their hearts. They also continue to support Jill in her much-needed work. Jill deeply misses her grandmother, and hopes she knew the impact she made in the talk they had one summer long ago.

When Jill began Aniridia Foundation International, it became a part of her. She puts her entire heart and soul into every aspect of it, which is why, when we speak of AFI, we are also speaking of Jill. They are one and the same, just as some say the holy trinity are one. Each and every day Jill continues to put herself into AFI, and is amazed to see all the accomplishments it has achieved in such a short time. In the beginning, it was very strenuous for Jill to start the foundation while raising her son, Michael, alone. She remembers him saying, "Can you get someone else to run this thing?" That is when she knew she had to get more help, make business hours, get a social life, and still keep her passion for the foundation. Jill says she was juggling and hoping the balls would stay in the air.

While raising Michael and starting the foundation she was struggling with going through five transplants and fifteen eye surgeries. She worried about finances, helping Michael at school (walking two miles to the school to get him and two miles back home with him since she couldn't drive), and riding a roller coaster of emotions from all the surgeries. Jill admits it was not easy, but she knew she *had* to keep going to make a difference for others with aniridia. She strongly believes, since not being able to go to medical school, that starting AFI was God's plan for her. He always gives her what she needs to continue her work while going through so many struggles.

Trying to work while going through the surgeries was quite grueling, since she could not see at times. While planning a medical conference in Wisconsin, Jill could barely see out of one eye because of corneal scarring. The doctor would not work on it until the glaucoma in her other eye was under control. Jill says this was the closest she has been to being completely blind, and she never wants to experience it again. But it did show her the importance of showing others how they could avoid blindness from corneal scarring. Working on the foundation kept her from worrying about things and dealing with her eyes' ups and downs. It kept Jill focused and made her recovery go well.

Throughout the years Jill has had many happy times where her vision and ptosis did not matter. But there were also times where people's misconceptions made her sad. Some people gave her positive remarks, such as that she had bedroom eyes, which was sexy. Yet others have made rude and not positive remarks because of the ptosis. Just a few examples of this are: not getting a job because the hiring manager thought she was stoned, having a man not want to talk to her at a party because he thought she was drunk when she never even had a drink, and having a waitress comment that Jill didn't need a drink because she looked like she'd already had enough when Jill had not had one drop of alcohol that day. Now when people comment that she looks tired, drunk, or stoned Jill simply says, "No, I'm not. I was born this way." Other times she may say, "I was born with an eye condition." Along with the public's perception, Jill has also struggled with not being able to drive. Going to get groceries could take up to three hours for her because she has to walk, since public transportation is not good in her area. It also frustrates her that she is not able to take Michael places he needs to go.

However, today Jill is thrilled that Aniridia Foundation International is continuing to grow rapidly and has members from all over the world. She feels there is strength in numbers, and knows that hope and excitement are contagious, which is why being a part of AFI has many advantages. Meeting others you can relate to helps you see you are not alone; gaining knowledge about aniridia and its associated conditions, and having experienced doctors available to answer questions are just two of the additional advantages. Jill and her fellow board members handpick each doctor who is on AFI's Medical Advisory Board. Jill wants to be sure each doctor is not only experienced in his or her specialty, but also has knowledge of aniridia. It is important to Jill to have doctors on AFI's Medical Advisory Board who are not only knowledgeable, but also give each patient the utmost care to preserve the patient's vision. Jill also feels that educating the public and medical communities will help those in the future who will be affected by aniridia. She first began AFI to help others like herself. Today her most important and ambitious goal is to stop aniridia from existing via genetic breakthroughs, or at least to stop its inheritance by the time she has to retire. If anyone can see this goal become a reality, it is Jill.

One way AFI unites people affected by aniridia worldwide is its website. The site is also a great way to gain information on aniridia. Some new things added to the website are a Physicians' Area and the ability to register donations online. In the near future, Jill hopes to add a web store to sell wristbands, T-shirts, infant/children sunglasses, and low-vision equipment. These things need a permanent webmaster with the knowledge to keep these additions up and running. Hopefully with some funding or a grant, AFI can hire at least one part-time individual to make these things happen.

Besides the website, AFI has a free quarterly members' newsletter with news about AFI, helpful information for members on such topics as employment issues, and many other subjects. It is a great way to keep up on the most recent AFI and medical information. In the beginning, Jill did the entire newsletter by herself. Then in 2004 several volunteers came together to help Jill with the newsletter, which is now called the *Eye on Aniridia*. A major goal of the newsletter is to give information to those who do not have a computer or Internet access. Jill would also like to find a way to start a phone support group so those with aniridia, and parents of children with aniridia, can talk to others who understand and can help answer questions.

In November 2005, AFI moved its offices to the Hamilton Eye Institute (HEI) in Memphis, Tennessee. Jill feels very privileged that the HEI is willing to help AFI in its fight against blindness. Jill is currently working on AFI's future goals. These goals are to educate and unite the aniridia population, put out some medical surveys to help researchers, and increase our knowledge of present treatments to find better ways to eliminate immune-suppression needs.

Jill knows she has a huge agenda, but believes that if you do not stretch for success you usually reach too low. That is why AFI has started its most significant program called the International Aniridia Medical Registry and Gene Bank. AFI is is collecting data from all those affected by aniridia. This registry is to educate doctors, get statistics, and help promote more research. It will also help educate doctors via clinical photographs so they can be better informed about aniridia and its associated conditions, treatments, and surgical procedures. To accomplish this, AFI is collecting DNA and tissue samples from those affect by aniridia along with their blood relatives. Once samples are collected, the DNA is analyzed and entered into files in the International Aniridia Medical Registry and Gene Bank. AFI encourages all affected by aniridia to participate in this program. For more information please call AFI's office, go to AFI's website at www.aniridia.net, or email info@aniridia.net. The information from these tests will be given to AFI and the patients who provide samples. All personal information on the registry and tests will be confidential. Jill is optimistic about this project because it is a stepping-stone in finding a way to stop aniridia.

Another important medical AFI program is the OPTIC (Ophthalmic PaTient Immunosuppression Clinic) Program. This program is to help those who have undergone KLAL surgery. This program is to ensure that patients have the best medical care, education, and monitoring possible. It is the beginning of further plans to open clinics at various institutions where KLAL procedures are being done and doctors are well trained in immunosuppression and the KLAL procedure. Plus, since AFI is compassionate to those who also experience blindness from corneal pannus, AFI wanted to create this program that would also help those affected by Stevens-Johnson syndrome and chemical and thermal burns to the eye.

AFI has several other programs and events. These successful ventures are CUDDLES, We Care, social gatherings, newsletters, physicians' and researchers' meetings, fundraising events, and medical conferences. Jill created CUDDLES for young children who have gone through transplants/surgeries. The children are given a personalized stuffed animal. Jill first got her inspiration for CUDDLES from her psychology degree. She thought that using a teddy bear or stuffed animal in play therapy might help relieve stress or fear from doctor appointments, surgeries, etc. Jill first used this technique with a young girl who did not want Dr. Holland to check her eyes. Jill suggested he check the girl's stuffed bunny's eyes first. While in the waiting area they played doctor with the bunny. It seemed to help the little girl, and she allowed Dr. Holland to check her eyes.

We Care is like CUDDLES except it is a program to help adults who are undergoing transplants or surgeries with social gatherings and medical conferences where people can get to know one other and gain helpful information. For example, at medical conferences and on AFI's members' area website, experts give suggestions about where to get VEP tests for children or what doctors specializes in certain areas, so parents may have the opportunity to find the right doctor for their child.

AFI holds a biannual "Make a Miracle" medical conference and social. Several nternational members have even begun to attend these conferences.. Some members have come from China, New Zealand, Norway, and several other countries. Doctors and researchers speakat the conferences, helping educate not only those affected by aniridia, but each other. Two international doctors from Sweden and Norway even attended and spoke at the 2005 conference. During the conference there is a special Physicians' and Researchers' Day where the doctors and researchers come together to hear each other speak and to learn from one another. At upcoming conferences, AFI plans to have more international members, doctors, and researchers attend. AFI has recently found that the PAX 6 gene plays a part in the development of not only the eyes, but also other parts of the body; therefore, AFI plans to include discussions and information on such things as: diabetes/glucose intolerance, autism spectrum disorders, Polycystic Ovary Syndrome (PCOS), and sleep disorders.

In addition to AFI's members' newsletter, AFI has a newsletter just for doctors and researchers, *Aniridia InSight*. It is used to raise awareness and educate the medical community. Physicians and researchers can also attend meetings held by AFI to hear from top doctors experienced with aniridia and its associated conditions. This helps doctors give their patients with aniridia the latest and best care possible. In addition, there is a "think tank" portion of the meeting where all doctors and researchers can share patient issues and current research with one another. This helps get everyone affected by aniridia closer to improved health care, more awareness, better medical education, and research towards AFI's ultimate goal of a cure for aniridia.

Another crucial AFI program is fundraising events. These events are not only held by AFI, but several families have raised funds for AFI by themselves. Some families sent a letter out to their family members and friends asking them to donate to AFI instead of giving gifts at their son's birthday party. Just by doing this they raised a good sum for AFI. At AFI's biannual medical conference and socials the foundation holds its' grand social event and fundraiser called "Make A

Miracle" charity dinner along with a silent auction, and raffle. In previous years this event has raised a substantial amount, which has helped AFIto continue and expand its efforts. Another successful event was held on August 5, 2006. The event was a charity screening of Disney's film *Step Up,* which was produced by an AFI member and parent of a child with aniridia. The screening and after party were held in Southampton, Long Island. Even some celebrities came to support the fundraising event. Carmen Electra and David Blaine, illusionist and endurance artist, were hosts of the event. At the after party the celebrity auction was very successful. One lucky bidder won a role in filmmaker Adam Shankman's movie *Hairspray.* Another bidder won a day of magic lessons with David Blaine. The event was so successful that it exceeded its goal. More and more members are stepping up by planning and hosting fundraisers for AFI. On August 2, 2008, one family in Illinois organized and hosted a candlelight bowl that sold out a bowling alley of 300 people and raised an amazing amount for AFI. On June 7, 2009 another family stepped up and chaired a new AFI annual fundraiser called "Songs for Sight." The event was held at Hersey Area Playhouse in Hersey, Pennsylvania, and had Steve Roslonek of SteveSongs (as seen on PBS Kids TV) perform. This event sold out in record time and raised a wonderful amount for AFI. Because of active member like these families, today AFI continues to exponentially grow in its membership and funds. It prides itself in providing its programs and events with little to no charge to its' members; however, for it to continue to do so it needs continual donations and volunteers.

If you would like to help keep hope alive, you can volunteer or donate to AFI. AFI has several committees it needs volunteers for, and just some of them are: fundraising, publicity, *Eye on Aniridia* members' newsletter staff, *Aniridia InSight* newsletter staff, offline communications/support groups, and many others. In a recent *Eye on Aniridia* article about AFI's future goals, Jill Nerby wrote, "We need volunteers to help us with their time or special talents, because volunteering is as important as financial contributions. Please be active! Be a part of the solution!" For more information on how you can volunteer, please e-mail us at info@aniridia.net. You can donate online at www.aniridia.net or call our office.

You can also go to your human resources department and find out if it belongs to the United Way Payroll Designated Deduction program. If the foundation is not on their list, it can be put on it if you fill out an application that the department needs to add the foundation to the list. AFI can have volunteers contact the different United Ways for information on how to be listed in their nonprofit lists. If you would like to become a member of AFI, please visit the website at www.aniridia.net.

Members of the AFI were asked, how has AFI helped and is AFI important to you? Below are just a few of the answers we received.

Without AFI I would feel lost without others who share the same eye condition as I do. I think it is important to talk to others and let go of frustration.

—Brittany

The last convention was a huge information overload that you can't get from anywhere else! It was wonderful to meet others just like my child, and we are looking forward to the next one.

—Christy

AFI is an important tool, not just for parents, but for schools' special education departments. Our school district has never heard of nor dealt with aniridia before, so our daughter will be their first and we are looking forward to working with them.

—Dawn

I think AFI helps a lot, because at least now I know that others have experienced the things I have gone through, to some extent. Before I knew about the foundation, I felt very alone and isolated. The people around me (except my father) didn't really understand what I was going through or how to help me.

—Rosemarie

Without AFI I would be more worried about how my son will handle the problems that will arise when he starts school and becomes a teenager. The foundation has allowed me to read stories of many successful and well-adjusted young people with aniridia. Plus, since there are very few doctors in the U.S.A. who are specialists in aniridia, AFI is a great way for us to hear about new research that can help individuals with aniridia.

—Elizabeth

It is very important and encouraging that AFI exists. Without such an organization the minority of people with aniridia struggling to succeed would truly have no voice and would be left completely in the dark.

—Matthew

AFI'S EXECUTIVE BOARD

Jill A. Nerby, Founder and CEO, Aniridia Foundation International, Hamilton Eye Institute, Memphis, Tennessee, U.S.A.

Edward Holland, M.D., Director of Cornea Services—Cincinnati Eye Institute, Professor of Ophthalmology—University of Cincinnati, Cincinnati, Ohio, U.S.A.

Peter A. Netland, M.D., Ph.D., Professor and Chairman—Department of Ophthalmology—University of Virginia School of Medicine, Charlottesville, U.S.A.

Christopher Albrecht, C.P.A., Ammon & Albrecht, C.P.A.s, Springboro, Ohio, U.S.A.

AFI'S MEDICAL ADVISORY BOARD

Aniridia Research

- John Crolla, Ph.D., MRCPath, Wessex Regional Genetics, United Kingdom.
- Ali Djalilian, M.D., Assistant Professor of Ophthalmology and Visual Sciences—University of Illinois, Chicago, Illinois, U.S.A.
- James Lauderdale, Ph.D., Associate Professor—University of Georgia, Athens, Georgia, U.S.A.
- Veronica van Heyningen, D.Phil, FRSE FmedSci, MRC Human Genetics Unit, Edinburgh, United Kingdom.

Corneal and External Disease

- Edward Holland, M.D., Director of Cornea Services—Cincinnati Eye Institute, Professor of Ophthalmology—University of Cincinnati, Cincinnati, Ohio, U.S.A.
- John Freeman, M.D., Memphis Eye and Cataract Associates, Memphis, Tennessee, U.S.A.

Counseling

Mark Pishotta, M.A., L.L.C., N.C.C., Chicago, Illinois, U.S.A.

Glaucoma

- Peter A. Netland, M.D., Ph.D., Professor and Chairman—Department of Ophthalmology—University of Virginia School of Medicine, Charlottesville, U.S.A.
- Lama Al-Aswad, M.D., Professor of Clinical Ophthalmology (Glaucoma Division) of the Harkness Eye Institute—Columbia University, New York, New York, U.S.A.

Glaucoma—Pediatric

- David Walton, M.D., Boston, Massachusetts, U.S.A.
- Anil Mandal, M.D., Director of Children's Eye Care Center, LV Prasad Eye Institute, India.

Genetics

- Eniko Pivnick, M.D., University of Tennessee, Memphis, Tennessee, U.S.A.
- Richard Lewis, M.D., M.S., Cullen Eye Institute—Baylor College of Medicine, Houston, Texas, U.S.A.

Vision Specialists/Teachers

- Cay Holbrook, Ph.D., University of British Columbia.

AFI's Scientific Board is currently be created and will be headed by co-chairs James Lauderdale, Ph.D., and Ali Djalilian, M.D.

The doctors on AFI's Medical Advisory Board are hand-picked. Each has extensive experience in aniridia and low vision. The goal is to have three to four national and international doctors for each category, so there is a diverse group with different points of views to discuss the best options for aniridia patients.

ANIRIDIA FOUNDATION INTERNATIONAL MISSION STATEMENT

Overall Goal: To cure aniridia and its associated conditions.

Immediate Goal: To help those affected by working to improve medical care and understanding, to raise funds for research projects that would help aniridia and its associated conditions, and to pursue better treatments and services to enable them to have a healthy, independent life.

Everyday Goal: To promote awareness among the public and medical community through educational and fund-raising programs, to dispel misconceptions, and finally, to pursue and unite people with aniridia to create a medical registry, which in turn will help us with our goals above to move forward in research and treatments, and closer to a cure. (*Jill Nerby, AFI Mission Statement*)

Through it all Jill continues to work hard and inspire all she meets. She keeps a positive attitude, and strongly believes:

- *If you believe in yourself you can do almost anything.*
- *Attain your goals: Work hard, pray harder, and believe you will have help in doing it.*
- *Do not let people's ignorance make you bitter or angry, but use it as energy to do something to increase awareness. Be a part of the solution, not the problem.*

UNITED, WE CAN MAKE A DIFFERENCE!

13

Other Support Services

JESSICA J. OTIS

Besides the support of Aniridia Foundation International, there are several other services for the blind and visually impaired. Parent Training and Information Centers and Community Parent Resource Centers can help parents with children who are blind or visually impaired. These centers are located all over the United States, and they help families of children and young adults with disabilities (from birth to age 22). Also, they help families obtain appropriate education and services for their children with disabilities, train and inform parents and professionals on a variety of topics, resolve problems between families and schools, and connect children with disabilities to community resources that address their needs. For more information on a center located in your state, please visit http://www. taalliance.org/centers/index.htm or visit http://www.ilru.org/html/publications/ directory/index.html.

All websites mentioned in this chapter will be listed at the end of this chapter along with several other websites for other services and organizations that may assist you.

LIGHTHOUSE INTERNATIONAL

The Lighthouse International has been helping visually impaired people since 1905. It strives to help visually impaired individuals live better lives and to be in independent. It is also dedicated to preventing disabilities. To accomplish this it has research studies, prevention efforts, advocacy initiatives, education programs, and vision rehabilitation services. For more information, please visit the Lighthouse International website at www.lighthouse.org.

LIONS INTERNATIONAL

The Lions International began to dedicate services to the visually impaired in 1925 when Helen Keller challenged the Lions Club to be "knights of the blind in the crusade against darkness." Today Lions is successful in helping those who are blind and visually impaired. A very important program Lions has is called SightFirst. This program was started in 1989 to help prevent blindness. Just a few of the services are helping to construct or expand eye hospitals and clinics, contributing to cataract surgeries, and providing sight-saving medication. This program is also striving to eliminate preventable childhood blindness, and to control river blindness and trachoma. For more information, please visit the Lions International website at www.lionsclubs.org.

AMERICAN FOUNDATION FOR THE BLIND

The American Foundation for the Blind (AFB) is dedicated to the vital issues of the blind and visually impaired (such as independent living, employment, technology, and literacy). Helen Keller devoted her life to the AFB to ensure that blind and visually impaired individuals have the same rights and opportunities that others have in this country. Miss Keller was a spokesperson for the AFB from 1924 until her death in 1968. Upon her death the AFB received her books, papers, photographs, and artifacts from her library. All of these items are a part of the Helen Keller Archives in New York City at the AFB's headquarters. Some the archives can be seen on the AFB's website at www.afb.org. The AFB maintains five national centers across the United States, and in Washington, D.C., it has a governmental relations office. A special program the AFB has is called the Braille Bug. It teaches children Braille and the importance of it. The AFB also has information for parents, professionals, and seniors. The organization is a strong advocate for ensuring that government programs and policies meet the needs of those who are blind or visually impaired, and their families. It focuses on federal and state programs that may affect the education and rehabilitation of those who are blind or visually impaired, and also on laws that relate to economic status and civil rights. For further information, please visit the AFB's website at www.afb.org.

FOUNDATION FOR THE JUNIOR BLIND

The Foundation for the Junior Blind (FJB) was founded in 1953 by Norman Kaplan to provide recreational services to children who are blind or visually impaired. Later in the 1960s, Henry Bloomfield gave the foundation property to establish a year-round camp in California for blind and visually impaired children and their families. Now it provides services to over 6,000 individuals every year in California and its neighboring states. The FJB's mission is to "provide services and programs for children and adults who are blind or visually impaired and their families to achieve independence and self-esteem."[1] Some of the programs that the FJB offers are Infant Family Program, Camp Bloomfield, Student Transition and Enrichment Program (STEP), and Visions-Adventures in Learning. The Infant Family Program "provides specialized in-home services for children who are multiply disabled-blind from birth through three years of age."[2] STEP is a recently established program that is for young people from 16 to 22 years old who are blind or visually impaired. It assists them in identifying their career interests and helps them learn skills necessary to achieve their career goals. Visions-Adventures in Learning gives new experiences to teens who are blind or visually impaired. Some things they may learn and build are self-esteem, a sense of teamwork, and overall personal growth. Camp Bloomfield has several activities for the children, such as swimming, hiking, horseback riding, wall-climbing activities, learning to help themselves by helping others, and learning about responsibility and leadership. For more information on Camp Bloomfield and the FJB, please visit the website at www.fjb.org.

NATIONAL FEDERATION OF THE BLIND

A major organization that helps the blind and visually impaired is the National Federation of the Blind (NFB). The NFB was founded in 1940 and is now the largest membership organization of the blind in the United States. It has 50,000 members and over 700 local and state chapters. The first important thing you should know about the NFB is that it is an organization "of" blind people, which means that the blind determine their own priorities and programs rather than someone else determining it for them. In addition, an important statement that the NFB uses often is, "The real problem of blindness is not the loss of eyesight. The real problem is the misunderstanding and lack of information which exists. If a blind person has proper training and opportunity, blindness is only a physical nuisance."[3] While the NFB is an organization "of" blind people, they do encourage individuals who are not blind to come and participate in the NFB's efforts. In fact, the NFB has many sighted members. The NFB's constitution requires the elected leaders, particularly the presidents, and the majority of the membership to be blind, but otherwise sighted individuals can fully participate in the organization.

Wanting to learn more about the NFB from someone who is very knowledge-able about it and works for the NFB, I talked to my good friend Mark Riccobono. Mark is the director of education programs at the National Federation of the Blind's Jernigan Institute. When asked what were some of the most important things someone should know about the NFB, and what it does for the blind and visually impaired, Mark said one important message from the NFB is, "Blindness is feared the most by society. It is even feared more than death or cancer. Yet, blindness itself is not a tragedy, since a blind person can still live a full, productive life. To achieve a full, productive life, a person needs to learn from successful blind individuals who have learned the techniques and built the confidence, and to achieve their dreams despite blindness. This message is the fabric of the NFB, where blind people share and work with other blind people. By doing this the NFB's state and local chapters make a critical difference."

Another major aspect of the NFB is its published materials. Mark says:

These publications are written by blind people, and are about topics and issues that are relevant to blind individuals. They give a powerful perspective to others who are blind. Since society constantly sends us negative messages about blindness, this literature helps us to remember that blindness does not make up everything that we are; it is simply one of many characteristics. Also, the publications include the NFB's flagship publication, the *Braille Monitor* (available in print, Braille, or on cassette); *Future Reflections* (available in print and on cassette), a publication for parents and educators; and the NFB's new online publication, "Voice of the Nation's Blind," which you can visit online at www.voiceofthenations blind.org. All of these are available via e-mail. The NFB also produces *Voice of the Diabetic*. Since diabetes is a leading cause of blindness, this is important. Furthermore, the publications are important because they present articles about current issues impacting the blind and articles about achievements of blind people.

A third important aspect of the NFB is its several services and programs for the blind and visually impaired. Some of them are public education, national conventions, the Jernigan Institute, the Material Center, the International Braille and Technology Center, a job line, and the NFB Newsline.

An important contribution of the NFB is its public education program. Mark stated, "With public education the NFB spends much time educating the general public about what blindness is and what it is not. This includes teaching people about the capabilities of blind people." The NFB is very dedicated to advocacy for the blind and visually impaired. On this matter, Mark continues, "These efforts range from working with individual blind people on Social Security disputes and cases of discrimination, to pursuing legal remedy for discrimination against an individual or group, to educating the Congress about important issues impacting the blind. This also happens at all levels: local, state, and national."

The NFB also holds annual national conventions. The NFB conventions are a great opportunity to learn about blindness and the types of opportunities and tools available. A NFB convention can draw better than 3,000 blind people from all over the country and many from around the world. Mark stated, "The only way to really understand the power of the convention is to experience it yourself." In addition, each state holds a convention, and the local chapters have monthly meetings, which can help you become more educated and involved in the NFB. To find information on your state NFB chapter, please visit http://www.nfb.org/localorg.htm and click on your state for its contact information.

Another service of the NFB is the Newsline. Newsline is a newspaper talking service that gives the blind all the text of national and local newspapers just by using a touchtone telephone. From this technology the NFB Jobline was created. It is a free telephone menu system of national employment listings and job openings. Also, the NFB has a wonderful Material Center that has over 1,100 pieces of literature on blindness, and 400 appliances and aids for the blind. The NFB has the International Braille and Technology Center, which is the largest in the world. It has the most complete evaluation and presentation center for speech and Braille technology used by the blind from around the world.

On January 30, 2004, the NFB had its grand opening of the Jernigan Institute for the blind. The Jernigan Institute is a unique training and research facility for the blind and visually impaired. Some of the institute's programs are education, employment and rehabilitation, seniors, mentoring, and technology. The Jernigan Institute plans to improve technology, teach Braille, reduce unemployment rates by improving employment opportunities, and provide services and resources for seniors. Additionally, the Jernigan Institute has begun a project called the National Center for Mentoring Excellence. This project is to develop a mentoring program for blind and visually impaired (ages 16 to 26) to improve the outcome of employment. Two states that will begin this project are New Jersey and Louisiana. Mark said, "This program essentially puts together the research and best practices of what NFB has done for over sixty years. Just like with any program of the NFB, this program will be open to anyone regardless of his/her membership in NFB. To use NFB services, you do not have to be a member." For more information on the National Center for Mentoring Excellence, please e-mail aphelps@nfb.org or call the Jernigan Institute at (410) 659-9314, extension 2295. Furthermore, if you are interested in an internship opportunity at the NFB Jernigan Institute, please contact Mark Riccobono, Executive Director at the Jernigan Institute, at (410) 659-9314, extension 2368, or e-mail mriccobono@nfb.org to learn about current and future opportunities.

Finally, when asked what is the most important message to take away from the NFB, Mark said, "If you have a visual impairment that prevents you from doing any significant daily activities with your vision, meaning you need to use non-visual techniques, whether you want to admit it or not you are blind. It is respectable to be blind. Furthermore, the best way to make your blindness into a positive experience that does not hold you back in any way is to interact with members of the NFB." If you would like more information or would like to join the NFB, please visit the website at www.nfb.org or contact your local chapter in your state.

Each of these organizations has valuable services, so take advantage by joining one or more so that you and your child may reap the rewards. For further information on each of these services and others, please see the following list of websites.

LIST OF SERVICES AND THEIR WEBSITES

AFB National Employment Listings—http://www.afb.org/Community.asp? Type=Employment

AFB Newsletter *Access World*—http://www.afb.org/aw/main.asp

American Foundation for the Blind (AFB)—www.afb.org

Aniridia Foundation International—www.aniridia.net

Blindness Related Resources—http://www.hicom.net/%7Eoedipus/blind.html

BryTech (technology for the blind and visually impaired)—http://www.brytech.com

Centers for Independent Living—http://www.ilru.org/html/publications/directory/index.html

Disability Info—http://www.disabilityinfo.gov

Foundation for the Junior Blind (FJB)—www.fjb.org

International WAGR Syndrome Association—http://www.wagr.org/index.html
Internet Resource for Special Children (IRSC)—http://www.irsc.org
Lighthouse International—www.lighthouse.org
Lions International—www.lionsclubs.org
Lions World Services for the Blind—http://www.lwsb.org
National Federation of the Blind (NFB)—www.nfb.org
NFB Local Chapters—http://www.nfb.org/localorg.htm
Office of Disability Employment (U.S. Dept. of Labor)—http://www.dol.gov/odep/
Parent Training and Information Centers and Community Parent Resource Centers—http://www.taalliance.org/centers/index.htm

Notes

1. Foundation of the Junior Blind, available: www.fjb.org, 2006.
2. Foundation of the Junior Blind, available: www.fjb.org, 2006.
3. National Federation of the Blind, available: www.nfb.org, 2006.

Appendix

Aniridia Foundation International Member
Emergency Information

Aniridia is a congenital eye condition causing partial or complete absence of the iris plus other ocular and medical conditions.

Name: _____

Address: _____ State: _____ Zip: _____

Country: _____

Phone# (_____)_____

Email: _____

Emergency Contact: _____

Contact's Phone # (_____)_____

Member's Relationship with Contact: _____

Member's Ophthalmologist: _____

Member's Ophthalmologist Phone # (____) _____

Member has: Familial ____ Sporadic ____ Aniridia

Other associated conditions:

_____

_____

Any other important information needed in case of an emergency:

_____

_____

_____

Member or Guardian's Signature:

_____

Glossary

abdomen: The cavity of the belly, containing the stomach, the intestines, and other organs.

abdominal: Of the abdomen.

allele: One member of a gene pair.

allograft (also known as allogeneic transplant or homograft): A transplant from a genetically non-identical member of the same species; most human transplants are of this type.

amblyopia: A condition in which the vision is decreased but no cause can be detected during eye examination.

amniotic fluid: Nourishing and protective liquid in the womb of a pregnant woman.

angle of the anterior chamber: That part of the eye between the cornea and the iris that drains the fluid within the eye out of the eye and maintains the pressure within the eye at normal levels.

aniridia: The congenital absence or partial absence of the iris. It usually carries with it other medical conditions.

anophthalmia: Complete absence of the eyes.

anterior: Nearer the front (opposite of "posterior").

aphakia: The absence of the lens of the eye.

aqueous humor: The liquid between the lens and the cornea. It is constantly made by a section of the ciliary body (the iris and the muscles around the lens).

astigmatism: Blurred vision due to incorrectly focused light (usually due to a damaged or misshapen cornea).

ataxia: Lack of coordination for movement.

atypical aniridia: The iris may appear normal, but is thinner than normal.

autosomal: Relating to chromosomes other than sex chromosomes.

avascular: Lacking blood vessels.

basal: Original.

basement membrane: A sheet of cells and fibers that covers the epithelium.

biconvex: Convex (curved outward) on both sides.

bilateral amblyopia: A reduction or dimness in vision.

181

bilateral aniridia: Aniridia in both eyes.

blepharitis: Inflammation of the eyelid.

bulbar conjunctiva (also called ocular conjunctiva): The part of the conjunctiva covering the eyeball.

cataract: An opacity of the lens in the eye that diminishes and can eventually eliminate the transparency of the lens required for vision.

CCTV: Acronym for closed circuit television.

cerebellum: The part of the brain that is responsible for maintaining muscle tone, balance, and coordination.

chorionic villus sampling (CVS): A method of prenatal diagnosis that tests placental tissue for genetic abnormalities.

ciliochoroidal detachment: An abnormal accumulation of serous fluid in the suprachoroidal space between the sclera externally and the choroid and ciliary body internally. This condition is often associated with hypotony, intraocular surgery, and inflammation. However, ciliochoroidal detachments can arise spontaneously or from an unknown cause.

cornea: The transparent layer that is the front of the eye.

choroid: The vascular layer between the retina and the sclera.

coloboma: A hole in an eye structure.

congenital: Being born with a genetic condition.

conjunctival: A transparent layer that covers the white of the eye (sclera) and the inside of the eyelids.

corneal epithelia: Clear cells that cover the surface of the cornea that are separated from the conjunctival by the corneoscleral limbus.

corneoscleral limbus: Where limbal stem cells are located, and become cornea epithelia cells.

cryptic deletion: A change in the chromosome that is not clearly understood.

cytogenetically detectable: Detectable through testing chromosomes (DNA).

cytogenetic deletion: Deletion of a whole chromosome or a segment of a chromosome.

cytokeratin: A protein present in epithelial tissue.

Descemet's membrane: Basement membrane between the stroma and the endothelial layer of the cornea. Endothelial cells require its support and cannot regenerate after injury without it.

de novo: Latin for "from the new"; a *de novo* mutation arises from a newly defective gene rather than a mutation passed down from a parent who already has that defective gene.

diabetes mellitus: Varying or persistent hyperglycemia (unusually high blood sugar), especially after eating.

diplopia: Double vision.

ectopia lentis: Displacement of the lens.

edema: Swelling.

emmetropic: The normal condition of the eye, with the refractive power of the cornea and the axial length of the eye correctly balanced so that objects are in sharp focus with the lens in a relaxed/neutral condition.

endocapsular ring: A surgical device that provides internal support for the capsular bag after and sometimes during phacoemulsification when zonules are missing or weak.

endophthalmitis: Inflammation of the internal coats of the eye.

epitheliopathy: A disease involving the cornea epithelium.

epithelium: Membranous tissue of one or more layers of cells.

EUA: Acronym for Examination Under Anesthesia.

explantation: Removal/transfer to a nutritive medium.

FISH analysis: Technique to detect chromosome mutations.

fluorescein: A yellow-green dye that fluoresces when illuminated with light of a specific wavelength. It can be applied directly to the cornea to detect cornea abnormalities.

fovea: The area of the retina that is responsible for the sharpest focused vision.

Gillespie syndrome: A rare genetic disorder that affects the eyes and brain. Symptoms can vary greatly, but in most reported cases patients have bilateral partial aniridia and cerebella ataxia.

glaucoma: An optic nerve disease involving narrowing of the field of vision due to loss of retinal ganglion cells.

goblet cell: A cup-shaped cell that secretes mucus.

gonadoblastoma: Cancer of the genitals.

hemorrhage: Bleeding.

haploinsufficiency: Condition where, due to mutation, one copy of a gene is not functional, while the other copy cannot produce enough protein by itself to perform its function.

haptic: Relating to sense of touch.

heterozygosity: Having two different alleles of a gene.

histopathology: Study of tissue, especially abnormal tissue resulting from disease.

homeostasis: Ability to adjust internal environment to achieve stability.

horizontal nystagmus: Eyes involuntarily move side to side (left to right).

hyperopic: Farsighted.

hyperphagia: Overeating.

hyphema: Blood in the anterior chamber of the eye.

hypoplasia: Underdevelopment or absence.

hypotony: Overly low intraocular pressure.

IEP: Acronym for Individualized Education Program.

iris: The colored part of the eye that surrounds the black pupil in the center of the eye.

iris coloboma: A rare eye condition in which the ocular fissure fails to close fully. This can affect all or some of the structures in the eye including the iris, lens, macula, and optic nerve. Coloboma can also be associated with microphthalmia (small eyes).

iris hypoplasia: Lacking an iris.

karyotype analysis: Method using dye to find changes in chromosomes.

keratopathy: When an eye has a cloudy and scarred cornea due to lack of limbal stem cells. It can be painful and can eventually cause blindness.

KLAL: Acronym for *cadaveric keratolimbal allograft*.

lens: In the eye, the transparent, biconvex organ that (along with the cornea) refracts light to be focused on the retina.

limbal: Pertaining to the limbus.

limbal ring: Dark ring around the outside of the iris.

limbus: Edge (for instance, the corneal *limbus* is the edge of the cornea).

macula: The yellow oval near the center of the retina; it contains the fovea.

mean: Average.

meibomian glands (AKA tarsal glands): Sebaceous glands at the rims of the eyelids. They secrete sebum, keeping the tear film from evaporating or spilling.

metalloproteinase: A proteinase with a metal atom at its active center.

microphakia: An abnormally small crystalline lens.

monocular: Having one eye.

mosaicism: A condition where some cells are normal and some cells are abnormal, with changes in the structure or number of chromosomes.

muscular incardination: Improper execution of a muscular function.

nucleotides: Compounds whose arrangement in specific pairs makes up genetic information within genes.

nystagmus: Constant and involuntary wobbling movement of the eyeball.

null point: The point at which eyes focus and nystagmus stops or slows down. Many unconsciously find their null point by turning or tilting their head.

oblique nystagmus: Eyes involuntarily move diagonally.

optic nerve: The structure transmitting visual information from the retina to the brain.

palisades of Vogt: Collection of corneal epithelial cells in ridge-like areas at the corneoscleral limbus.

palpate (also palpation): To feeling or push on parts of the body to check for medical conditions.

pancreas: The abdominal organ that secretes insulin.

pancreatitis: Inflammation of the pancreas.

pannus: The flap formed over the cornea when blood vessels grow over it.

panocular: Affecting different parts of the eye.

PAX (gene): Paired box genes.

phacoemulsification: A form of cataract surgery where the eye's lens is emulsified with an ultrasonic hand-piece and aspirated from the eye; aspirated fluids are replaced with a balanced saline solution to maintain the shape of the anterior chamber.

Peter's anomaly: A rare form of anterior segment dysgenesis featuring abnormal cleavage of the anterior chamber.

phakic: Having the lens.

photophobia: Abnormal intolerance of light that can cause discomfort and pain.

PPCD: Acronym for Preschool Program for Children with Disabilities.

proteinase (AKA protease): A protein-cleaving enzyme.

ptosis: Droopy eyelids. The eyes do this to protect themselves from glare or bright light.

retina: Light-sensitive tissue covering the inner eye.

Riegers' Anomaly syndrome: A genetic eye condition; a malformation of the front of the eye between the cornea and the lens. Thus, the retina and optic nerve are rarely affected.

rotary/circular nystagmus: Eyes involuntarily move in a circle.

sporadic: Being born with a condition when neither parent exhibits the condition. No family history.

squamous: Resembling scales.

stem cells: Cells able to renew themselves via mitotic division and take on a variety of forms depending on context; the body's self-repair system.

strabismus: Squint, cross-eyes or wall-eyes.

stratified: Arranged in layers (strata).

stroma: Support tissue.

subluxation: Dislocation, displacement from normal position.

trabecular meshwork: Area between the cornea and the iris that drains away the aqueous humor.

trabeculectomy: Removal of trabecular meshwork to relieve intraocular pressure.

vertical nystagmus: Eyes involuntarily move up and down.

vitrectomy: Removal of vitreous humor from the eye.

vitreous humor (or just "vitreous"): Transparent gel filling the space between the lens and the retina.

WAGR syndrome: A rare genetic disorder. It stands for Wilms' tumor/Aniridia/Genitourinary abnormalities/Retardation.

Wilms' tumor: A type of malignant kidney tumor.

zonule (AKA "zonule of Zinn"): Ring connecting the ciliary body and the lens.

Index